T0339503

INTELLIGENT DRUG PRESCRIBING IN PSYCHIATRY

This new book, drawing on the author's distinguished career in front-line psychiatric practice, describes how to bring patient and prescriber together in an active partnership whereby there is better understanding of the positive and negative elements of drug prescription. At present there is a gap between expectations, with doctors not always able to admit their ignorance of some aspects of drug action, and patients kept unaware of these uncertainties. Balanced decision-making with joint involvement is needed to separate those drugs that are needed regularly to maintain health, those that are only needed when required, and those that are mere fashion accessories. Greater care is needed over the explanation of the first prescription, the expected duration of treatment and the plans for eventual withdrawal. The consequence of a better partnership will be less over-prescribing, a reduction of polypharmacy and a lessened need for deprescribing, the planned systematic reduction of drug treatment that has got completely out of control.

Concentrating on routine prescribing for psychiatric and mental health disorders rather than unusual conditions and illustrated with real-life anecdotes and case histories, this is essential reading for trainee and practising psychiatrics, general practitioners and pharmacists.

INTELLIGENT DRUG PRESCRIBING IN PSYCHIATRY

Supporting the Patient–Prescriber Partnership

Peter Tyrer
Emeritus Professor of Community Psychiatry
Division of Psychiatry
Imperial College London, UK
and
Visiting Professor of Psychiatry
Nottingham Trent University
Nottingham, UK

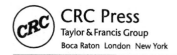

CRC Press
Taylor & Francis Group
Boca Raton London New York

CRC Press is an imprint of the
Taylor & Francis Group, an **informa** business

Designed cover image: Eoneren. iStock by Getty Images.

First edition published 2025

by CRC Press

2385 NW Executive Center Drive, Suite 320, Boca Raton, FL 33431

and by CRC Press

4 Park Square, Milton Park, Abingdon, Oxon, OX14 4RN

CRC Press is an imprint of Taylor & Francis Group, LLC

© 2025 Peter Tyrer

ISBN: 978-1-032-61900-2 (hbk)
ISBN: 978-1-032-60980-5 (pbk)
ISBN: 978-1-032-61901-9 (ebk)

DOI: 10.1201/9781032619019

Typeset in Bembo
by Apex CoVantage, LLC

DEDICATION

Dedicated to Maria, Leroy and all other patients
who are breaking the barriers that prevent good
prescribing practice.

CONTENTS

PREFACE

This book has been written out of frustration. We live in an age of open dialogue, one in which we no longer hide behind barriers that inhibit communication and in which the restrictions of the words 'need to know' are recognised to be hollow excuses. Yet there is still a feeling among many practitioners that when it comes to the prescribing of drugs, the less said the better. The view becomes, 'explaining how drugs work will only confuse; this is one area where doctor knows best and the patient has to accept it'.

But in the case of drugs used for mental illness, doctors very rarely know best, and when they, and everybody else, are ignorant of the wide deserts of our understanding, we, the patients, ought to be aware of this. The aim of this book is to marry the scepticism of drug usage by those who are critical, exemplified by Joanna Moncrieff (2020), with the enthusiasm of those who advocate their use, well illustrated by David Nutt (2021, 2023), whose major interest at present is in expanding the use of psychedelic drugs. The sceptics and enthusiasts seldom meet, only tossing barbs at each other occasionally in the coded language of learned journals, but this is not the way forward.

I was hoping that both Joanna and David could give endorsements to this book, but I only have one, from David. Joanna felt she could not give support as she feels I have oversimplified her arguments supporting the drug-centred model. I am sorry I have failed to convince her, but I hope the reader will note that on many occasions, I quote her wise words in debunking common misperceptions and am sure she will defend herself elsewhere.

The patient–prescriber partnership might be an over-used phrase, but when it is properly exercised, it represents genuine understanding – an equal representation of knowledge and ignorance that leads to both parties' being in tune and comfortable with whatever follows the first prescription. A good prescriber is like a favourite walking stick, always keeping you in step and supporting when you stumble.

This book does not go into the details of specific drugs, although the last chapter lists each one and its dosage range. For the full account of the nature of each individual drug, and the strategies of both prescription and withdrawal, the Maudsley Guidelines cannot be surpassed (Taylor et al., 2021; Horowitz & Taylor, 2024), but please note that pharmacology should not be our only guide; patients can provide their own secret ingredients to make it succeed.

Peter Tyrer

AUTHOR

Peter Tyrer is Emeritus Professor of Community Psychiatry in the Division of Psychiatry at Imperial College, London, UK and Visiting Professor of Psychiatry at Nottingham Trent University, Nottingham, UK. His main research interests are models of delivering community psychiatric services, the classification and treatment of common mental illnesses, particularly anxiety and health anxiety, and the classification and management of personality disorders. He also leads research on the management of patients with intellectual disability and on new psychological treatments for a common but largely unrecognised condition, health anxiety. He is experienced in the management of those with severe mental illness, substance misuse and personality disorder and has developed a new treatment, nidotherapy, to help these people by making environmental, not personal, changes. Much of his recent work has been concerned with improving and extending the concept of personality disorder. Personality disturbance is very common not just in psychiatric practice, and this importance has been largely unrecognised as the classification system for this group of disorders is so poor. Fortunately, a major reform of classification has been agreed upon in the 11th revision of the International Classification of Diseases that we hope will destigmatise a very common form of mental distress.

INTRODUCTION

Prescription drugs are big business; they cost £9.69 billion in the United Kingdom in 2022. A significant proportion of the total was spent on psychotropic drugs (psychotropic is the term used to describe all drugs primarily used for mental disorders). Just to give a flavour of the costs involved, 83 million prescriptions were for antidepressants (£247 million), 13 million for antipsychotic drugs (£125 million) and 14 million for hypnotics and anti-anxiety drugs (£101 million). This book aims to achieve a reduction in these totals, particularly for the two biggest groups, as my experience, and that of many others, suggests that too many drugs are being prescribed inappropriately and unwisely. Part of the reason for this is that patients and prescribers do not always have a mutually reinforcing relationship: when they do, a more rational prescribing partnership is almost certainly created.

I am writing this book as a practitioner who has been both prescribing and recommending the prescription of psychotropic drugs by others ever since 1965 when I first qualified. In my first post, I had to see psychiatric as well as medical patients and recall that there were only a few drugs available at that time. I well remember having an impassioned argument with a senior medical colleague who would not allow a barbiturate to be given to an extremely agitated patient because he was afraid she would have a respiratory arrest and die. My argument was that she was suffering so much from agitation that a small dose of a barbiturate would take the edge of her anxiety and do no harm. Even now I am not sure who was right.

My other reason for writing this book was to correct much of the over-simplified thinking about these drugs. Much of the criticism comes from patients who feel they have not been given enough information

DOI: 10.1201/9781032619019-1

about the drugs they have been prescribed and regret ever taking them. But they are also being backed up by critics with more expertise who are increasingly taking the view that the benefits of most psychiatric drugs are greatly overstated, that the scientific justification of their use is based on false premises, and that most are basically useless. These critics have a point, the science of psychopharmacology has been a little smug in its attitudes, and its practitioners have been at fault in not paying more attention to the adverse effects of drugs, but that is not the whole story. Without drugs in psychiatry, we would have much more suffering and many more patients in hospitals and other institutions.

In this book, I am trying to achieve a balance between the extremes of the critics who cry havoc and oppose all those who promote drug treatment and the enthusiasts who have always believed that in time the psychopharmacological revolution will end the misery of mental illness without the need for complicated talk. The wider the menu of treatments in psychiatry the better; we just need more joint choices in practice.

I start this with a personal story that may seem irrelevant, but it has a message. In 1958, I attended an admission interview for an undergraduate place at Gonville & Caius College, Cambridge. This has been well known as the most medical of Cambridge colleges since the time of William Harvey, who first described the circulation of blood in the body. When I walked into the interview room, it appeared I was being interviewed only by the senior tutor. During the course of questioning I, after the first few minutes, became aware of a half-hidden second figure, relaxed and recumbent, or possibly asleep, on a sofa in the far corner of the room. This awakened a vague recollection that I was also going to be interviewed by someone called 'the pastor', so perhaps this was something to do with mentoring of undergraduates.

The senior tutor interviewed me in a correct and conventional manner, and I gradually lost interest in the distraction at the edge of the room. Then came the predictable question, 'What branch of medicine would you wish to pursue were you to be successful in coming here?' At last, an easy question. 'Psychiatry', I promptly responded. There was a pregnant silence. The senior tutor struggled for something intelligent to say. Suddenly a disembodied voice rose from the sofa; 'What would you do with people; speed them up or slow them down?' 'I think the subject is a complex one', I replied, desperate not to continue this line of conversation, 'but on balance I would be inclined to slow them down'. The owner of the voice appeared satisfied and drifted back into oblivion.

After my interview, I discovered that 'the pastor' was actually the Master of the College, Sir James Chadwick. He won the Nobel Prize in physics for his discovery of the neutron. He also played a major role as one of the few British scientists to be closely involved with Robert Oppenheimer in the Manhattan project that led to the development of the atomic bomb. It would be wrong of me to necessarily assume that he was thinking of psychiatry in the same way as particle physics, with electrons circulating around atoms, but something of this general nature must have generated his question.

This was hardly an irrelevant question and could be regarded as central to this book. Are psychiatrists just slowing over-active and excited people and speeding them up when they slow down? Joanna Moncrieff, one of the most trenchant critics of the overinclusive hypotheses of many psychopharmacologists, sums up the action of most psychiatric drugs in exactly these words. 'Drugs are not a sophisticated way of restoring or enhancing normal functioning. They are just drugs. They can temporarily speed you up or slow you down' (Moncrieff, 2020, pp. 179–180).

So Joanna and James, critical psychiatrist and Nobel Prize-winner, were on the same page. Both the particle circling around the atomic nucleus and the drug circling a nuclear syndrome have close affinity. But this book, starting with the first chapter, hopes to show that Joanna's hypothesis is to some extent wrong and over-simplified. The relationship between prescriber and patient will go nowhere if all we talk about is uppers and downers or summarise all of them as 'just drugs'.

This book is written to help readers, both mental health professionals and informed members of the public, to better understand the drugs used in the treatment of mental illness and to share this understanding easily. The reasons why better sharing is not easy to come by are a direct consequence of conflicting messages from 'experts', a word placed in quote marks because their expertise does not always apply to the forms of communication they use, and patients, who want to ask important questions but do not get a chance to do so. Prescribers should be experts in the area in which they practise, and the patients they treat should respect them for their expertise. This cannot be achieved if one group is perpetually decrying the use of drugs and another is embracing them too enthusiastically. There is a need for better balance.

The stimulus for this book came from a patient I was seeing for nidotherapy. Nidotherapy, or nest therapy, is the collaborative and systematic adjustment of the environment to improve mental health and is particularly focused on those with long-term mental health and personality problems. It was first described 22 years ago (Tyrer, 2002) and may seem far separated from drug treatment, but an encounter in 2012 changed all that.

Maria was a patient who attended one of our annual nidotherapy workshops that year. She had suffered from bipolar disorder for 20 years and over the course of this time had received many psychotropic drugs, mainly from the antipsychotic group. She had also had four admissions to hospital, precipitated by her disorder. Like many patients with recurring illness, she had learnt a lot about its manifestations over the years. In particular, she had the ability, gratifyingly present in a small number of patients with psychotic illness, to identify the warning signs of relapse, either to hypomania (elevated mood) or to depression, in advance of the main symptoms. She was therefore able to adjust her medication to anticipate the changes and help to offset a sudden elevation or reduction of mood.

Unfortunately, as is common practice in those with psychotic disorders, her regular medication was prescribed in fixed dosages at specific times of day. By taking more or less than prescribed, she fell afoul of her psychiatrist, who at first thought she was an unreliable pill taker. It took many months for her to persuade him that she was a diligent monitor of her drug consumption, but with time, she has managed to persuade him and others that she can be trusted to use her medication wisely. As a consequence, her total consumption of drugs has fallen, and she has fewer side effects. Maria has continued to press for a better interaction between patient and doctor so that flexibility of drug administration can become the norm rather than the exception. Maria has continued to attend the workshops of our charity – NIDUS-UK – and is keen to set up a group of like-minded people to promote her ideas.

This is just one example, but it is being replicated in many other patient–therapist interactions. The information explosion created by the Internet and social media has led to people knowing much more about medicines than their predecessors. No longer can doctors take refuge in empty statements such as 'you have a depression; these pills will take your depression away', 'your brain has become over-excited and needs to be calmed down' and 'you have a nervous condition that needs medication to get it back in order'. Armed with printouts from Google about almost every named disorder, patients are prepared to joust with doctors when they come to their appointments, and woe betide loose talk and weak explanations. Patients now see doctors on a more equal footing. If they get a chance to speak, they want to know the likely speed of response and side effects of each drug both immediate and delayed, as well as asking about its mode of action. Comprehensive answers to these questions can seldom be given, and doctors have to be more confident in acknowledging their ignorance of subjects where no firm answers are forthcoming.

Intelligent prescribing involves an open and honest dialogue between patient, doctors and carers, so that decisions about treatment become consensual. But we cannot escape the sad fact that there are many occasions when drug therapy still has to be given under coercion. The reasons for this are complex and mainly depend on the disorder concerned and whether the patient has the mental capacity to engage in a constructive dialogue. But even in situations when medication is given compulsorily, there is no reason why at a later stage it could not be taken voluntarily. Ideally this should lead to a harmonious relationship with the patient's full acceptance and agreement to take the drugs prescribed. I acknowledge this cannot happen in every case, but the effort is still worthwhile.

To illustrate the core principles of this book, I am going to start with a conversation whose essential errors I have heard many times before, much more frequently in the distant past than now, between a patient and a doctor. In the past, the only professionals who could prescribe drugs were doctors, but now nurses and other specialists can prescribe, hence the frequent use of 'prescriber' rather than 'doctor' in this book.

The patient is Maureen, a woman aged 72 who has been persuaded by her two sons to seek advice for a belief she has that seems to make little sense to them.

Doctor:	What seems to be the problem, Mrs X?
Maureen:	*(Nervously)* I think I'm being watched.
Doctor:	Yes I know, but we're all being watched in some way. Who is watching you?
Maureen:	I don't know. It might be the devil. He seems to be in the house all the time. He looks like a shadow but I can watch his lips move and they are saying things like "your time has come".
Doctor:	Come off it. You don't really believe in devils do you? I think your mind is just playing tricks with you.
Maureen:	*(Taken aback)* But I think it must be the devil because every time he appears I feel he wants me. In the night I get so depressed when I see him and think if I go off to sleep I may wake up in Hell.
Doctor:	So you're not sleeping?
Maureen:	No, I'm full of dread, waiting to see him, so I can't relax and am awake most of the night.
Doctor:	It's clear to me that you are very short of sleep. Isn't that right?
Maureen:	Yes, but what can I do about the devil?
Doctor:	It seems clear to me that you need to shake off all these funny ideas about the devil by having a good night's sleep. Have you ever taken sleeping tablets before?

Maureen: No I haven't, I've never needed them.

Doctor: Well you need them now. Here's a prescription. Take the tablets every night an hour before you go to bed and once you get a good night's sleep all these funny ideas will go away. I'll see you again in three weeks.

Maureen: Are there any other effects I should know about?

Doctor: No, don't you worry about them. When you get your prescription, you'll be given a leaflet about side effects – just the usual things, tummy upsets and all that. No need to worry. So that's all. I look forward to seeing you again in three weeks.

What is wrong with this conversation? If we break it down, we have four slips in this conversation that prevent good understanding: rudeness, dismissiveness, impatience and arrogance. Even in the shortest of interviews, there needs to be some element of general introduction and enquiry that can facilitate the patient's presentation of the problem. Barging straight in is not right.

When the patient does have the courage to mention her worry, her hallucination, her delusion about the devil, whatever interpretation you wish to make, it needs to be explored by the doctor. But he is immediately dismissive, giving the impression that he doesn't believe what she is saying or she is completely misinterpreting her experiences; he fails to allow her to describe her beliefs and perceptions so he has no understanding of what her experiences are and why they are so troubling. He is impatient to get to a simple problem that he understands, and when she mentions her problem with sleep, his mind clicks into gear. 'Good, insomnia is a prominent subject in my medical dictionary that I know how to deal with'. His arrogance is shown by the premature conclusion that all her problems can be explained by sleep disturbance and she therefore only needs a hypnotic drug to get things right. An average GP consultation is only six minutes long, but a first interview has to be longer, and no excuse can be made for this summary guillotine of a complex problem. This subject will be visited again later in the book to show how this interview could be carried out much more constructively.

These comments about coercive prescribing show that the idea of a common partnership between patient and prescriber is not always possible. There is much less discussion about conditions such as marked intellectual disability and dementia in this book as the patient–prescriber relationship has to be carried out at arm's length with other personnel, be they professional carers, relatives or friends. For instance, the decision to prescribe drugs in children falls mostly on parents, but it is still possible for children to be very clear about the reasons for drug prescription and the expected effects.

In the most severe mental disorders, particularly when violent behaviour is shown, drugs often have to be given in emergency, usually by injection, a process now called rapid tranquillization. But the policy in managing violent and disruptive behaviour and in major psychoses is always to defuse difficult situations and get consensual treatment wherever possible (Pratt et al., 2023), and this is where experience of good collaborative management can be valuable.

Because intelligent prescribing requires both doctor and patient to have a basic knowledge of pharmacology and, increasingly, of the science of pharmacokinetics too, the first four chapters of this book describe both the theories of drug action and the likely mechanisms of their effects as they are absorbed, distributed and eventually cleared from the body. I have tried to make the descriptions here as understandable as possible for lay readers but still apologise for some of the jargon that is almost impossible to avoid.

There is one matter that does need to be cleared up right at the beginning, the notion of drugs restoring 'chemical balance. Joanna Moncrieff has a very clear view on this subject,

> the increased use of psychiatric drugs has come about partly because people have been convinced that mental health problems are caused by a 'chemical imbalance' and that a drug is required to put this right. This idea has been heavily promoted by the pharmaceutical industry and by official bodies like the American Psychiatric Association and the UK's Royal College of Psychiatrists, even though there is no good evidence that any mental disorder is produced in this way.
>
> (p. 10)

She extends this argument by adding, 'It is still regularly argued that, because drugs have biochemical effects, and because they appear to benefit people with psychiatric symptoms, at least in some instances, the disorder must be the result of a biochemical state that is the opposite to that produced by the drugs' (Moncrieff, 2020, p. 23).

I think Joanna has overstated this issue, but she is right in saying that we have no scientific evidence of biochemical 'imbalance' in our body chemistry being a cause of mental illness and we should stop using this term. But we can state that the concentrations of some important chemical substances in our bodies – dopamine, adrenaline, noradrenaline, acetylcholine – are altered greatly by drug treatment, and these probably, I repeat probably, give some idea of why the drugs are effective. But as with all science in progress, we are still remarkably ignorant of the exact mechanism by which drugs help in mental illness. It is not by restoring balance, it is not replacing a missing chemical in our brains and it is not a regenerator of substances that have been lost since early development. When used in the most effective way, they treat illnesses of limited duration in the same way that a crutch helps in limb injury: they allow much of normal function to continue while the natural processes of repair are taking shape, and, once the injury is better, the crutch is no longer necessary.

The real dilemmas are with long-term treatment. Can drugs act as long-term crutches when mental illness is known to be persistent, or should they be withdrawn? This is one of the most important puzzles in psychiatry, and nobody can pronounce on this with full authority.

This book is designed to make the prescription of psychotropic drugs a more even joint process, one in which prescribers, many of whom are now nurses, explain the purpose and actions of drugs in simple language, encourage questions from patients and strike a good balance between explaining benefits and listing risks. The consequence will be that better-informed patients will take their drugs more appropriately, be less likely to stop them prematurely and know much more about the changes to make when things do not run smoothly. For those who want to see the evidence for some of the statements I make, there is a full list of references at the end of the book. Many of these can be accessed through PubMed, the resource provided free by the National Library of Medicine in the United States. I have also added references to my own work, fairly liberally, in the text. This is not just showing off, though there is an element of that too: because I have had some influence on much of the work described in the book, any criticisms should be directed at me rather than to other authors. I also include references from older publications that illustrate now much prescribing has changed in the last 50 years.

As a final comment, I have no financial declaration of interest to report and have no connection with any pharmaceutical organisation, but I am the chair of the charity NIDUS-UK, where all the proceeds of sales of this book will be deposited, so I am a product champion for nidotherapy (which gets only the odd mention in this book). But product champions are well known for over-selling, and so this should be noted.

1

MODELS OF DRUG ACTION IN PSYCHIATRY

I start with a description of two conflicting models of the way drugs work in psychiatry, both of which, in their raw form, are wrong. Why is this relevant in this book? It is because both of these are held by large numbers of people, many of them patients or prospective patients, and as they are the main users of drugs, they merit our attention. I also add a brief history of drug treatment for mental illness as this partly explains the development of the two models. Neither of these models is correct, but because they are held by so many people, they have to be exposed for what they are: over-simplified views of a complex problem that hinder the relationship between prescriber and patient. The two approaches are described as the drug–centred model and the disease–centred model (Table 1.1).

These two very different views about the nature of drug action are incompatible, and each is so dismissive of the other that useful dialogue does not take place; as the views are so opposed, debates about them often end in anger. Both views are sincerely held but in the present state of our knowledge are simply wrong. Psychiatrists tend to adopt the disease-centred model, but many patients adopt the drug-centred one. Joanna Moncrieff feels the balance is wrong – 'because the drug-centred model of drug action clashes with the disease model it is wilfully ignored by mainstream psychiatry' (p. 178) – so I have given it more prominence here.

The history of drug treatment in psychiatry is a short one. Before the 1950s, the hypothesis that drugs speed you up or slow you down was accurate. We had amphetamine to speed you up and chloral and barbiturates to slow you down. Then the antipsychotic drug chlorpromazine appeared in 1950. It was sedative, like the barbiturates,

DOI: 10.1201/9781032619019-2

Table 1.1 Differences between the Two Main Models of Psychotropic Drug Use

Quality	Drug-centred model	Disease-centred model
Mechanism	Drugs speed people up or slow them down	Drugs act on disease receptors in the body to produce predictable effects
Specificity	There are few differences between speeding and slowing drugs apart from their adverse effects	Drugs are prescribed to treat specific mental diseases
Nature of action	Drugs do not correct chemical imbalance but interfere with normal function	The specific properties of a drug make them suitable for correcting identifiable pathology in the brain
Value	The positive effects of drug treatment are small and largely discounted by their adverse effects both in treatment and during withdrawal	An effective drug brings an ill person back to normal function by correcting brain abnormalities
Benefit	The massive increase in psychotropic drug prescription has had no positive effects on mental health	Drugs are valuable in psychiatry and have helped to improve mental health

but also had separate effects on behaviour and, before long, it was found to be effective in the treatment of schizophrenia and other severe mental illness.

This was followed by an explosion of interest from pharmaceutical companies, and within a few years there were dozens of new drugs available. This was dubbed 'the psychopharmacological revolution', and many argued that the reduction of beds in mental hospitals that began in the 1950s was a direct consequence of the benefit of these new drugs. These new drugs were not being synthesised in a vacuum: basic science was behind their introduction, and Nobel Prizes were awarded to those who showed the mechanisms of drug action. It is at this point that the old drug–centred model lost its way; it was overtaken by science.

A. MECHANISM

All those involved in drug treatment of mental illness can embrace the statement 'some drugs are sedating, others are stimulants'. The drug-centred model views this as a single dimension extending from drugs that can lead to unconsciousness or death when the sedation is massive to others such as amphetamines that can lead to over-excitement. The disease model is more nuanced. It allows drugs to have both stimulating and sedative properties, and it acknowledges that some drugs, notably alcohol, are sedative but nevertheless appear to be stimulants to those taking them. The disease model also has an explanation for this; it can be explained by the pharmacological properties of the drugs concerned. Alcohol stimulates the release of dopamine from the brain, and as dopamine is a chemical messenger (a neurotransmitter) that provokes increased activity and pleasure it is stimulating. At the same time, alcohol depresses activity in the nervous system and so is sedating, and everybody who has ever taken alcohol will recognise that these sedative and stimulating properties are closely related to time and dosage, provoking 'the desire but taking away the performance' of a wider range than Shakespeare's focus in his famous quotation.

B. SPECIFICITY

There are significant differences between the two models here. The drug-centred model sees very little specificity. It perceives drugs as like sets of stimulant and sedative weights, ranging from the calming touch of an antihistamine (e.g. Benadryl®) to the other extreme of intravenous amphetamine administered by drug abusers to achieve a 'high'. There are lots of drugs in between, but their distinctions are all based on sedation and stimulation to different degrees and often in combination. These drugs lack all sophistication; the patient could more or less take any of these at random to produce the desired effects.

The disease model, in its simplest form, states that each mental disease has a specific pathology and that drugs are focused on the management of that disease. The notion of the silver bullet, a single solution to a specific problem, is the ideal answer for each condition. As there are many disorders in psychiatry, there have to be many drugs to treat them. Currently, more than 80 different drugs are approved for prescription in the United Kingdom, separated into antidepressants, anti-anxiety medications, stimulants, antipsychotics and mood stabilisers, with some smaller extras (see Chapters 6 and 13). The disease model argues that each has a place in treatment and so contradicts the drug-centred model as only having a handful of possibilities.

C. NATURE OF ACTION

A drug is a foreign substance that when inserted into the body changes normal bodily function. So says the drug-centred model baldly and bluntly. In a few people, the change may be beneficial, but when the drug is withdrawn, it can take time for the body to adjust to being normal again. It is therefore not surprising that people get withdrawal symptoms at this time. Getting back to normal is not easy.

The disease model argues that each mental disease has its own pharmacological deficiencies. Drugs correct these by counteracting these deficiencies and so bring the person back to a more normal state. Each disease has its own deficiencies, so different drugs are needed for each one, and careful adjustment of dosage is needed to get the balance right.

D. VALUE

Drugs are of limited value, the drug-centred model says, with only slight benefit and multiple harms. One of the strongest critics of medication is Peter Breggin from the United States, who gives a blanket rebuttal of drug value, even ignoring the views of patients who claim they have been helped by medication:

> *Every class of psychiatric drugs – antidepressants, stimulants, tranquilisers, mood, stabilisers, and antipsychotics – causes mental impairments that often go unrecognised by the victim, even when they are severe. This misleads medicated patients into believing that they are doing better even when they're getting worse. As a result, people often feel they cannot live without psychiatric drugs when a careful history reveals that their lives have deteriorated during the time that they have been exposed to them.*

(Breggin & Cohen, 2007)

I cannot let this comment go have; it suggests patients are just dupes and their minds so addled by medication they have ceased to function properly. This completely devalues the patient's voice. It is best answered by Linda Gask, a professor of psychiatry who has written eloquently about her experience of depression. 'It is difficult to comprehend why so many people want to prove antidepressants to be ineffective when my personal perception is that I wouldn't still be here without them. What is that saying about me and my lived experience?' (Linda Gask, tweet 16th June, 2021 (linda Gask, X), July, 2021).

The disease model regards drugs in the same way as physicians look at many medical illnesses, particularly chronic ones. A condition such as arthritis (both rheumatoid and osteoarthritic forms) is treated with drugs to relieve symptoms (pain) but also to combat inflammation (steroids) and correct some of the manifestations of the disease. Therefore, an antidepressant can not only be calming and reduce agitation but also, in the longer term, corrective of the mood disturbance by its pharmacological action.

BENEFITS

The benefits of drug therapy are minimal, if present at all, according to the drug-centred model. Each drug administered interferes with the whole body and so is associated with often unpleasant side effects, and any benefit achieved may be offset by the problems of withdrawal when the drug is stopped. It may not even be possible to stop the drug entirely because of withdrawal effects. So overall the range of benefits extends from slight improvement only in the short term to significantly worse over time.

The disease model maintains that when the right drug is chosen for the right disease there is a marked improvement and that this far outweighs any side effects or withdrawal problems.

WHICH MODEL SHOULD BE CHOSEN?

Both these models suffer from serious error. The drug-centred model provides a grossly oversimplified view of drug action, suggesting that all drugs lack sophistication and bludgeon the psyche rather like hammer blows attempting to correct the delicate functioning of a watch. The model was partly true until the end of the 19th century, as the few drugs available (opium and herbal remedies) were unselective and replete with unpleasant after-effects. It would be quite wrong to assume that the many psychoactive drugs available today are essentially the same.

The disease model does not stand up when compared with the equivalent of medical diseases. A mental disorder does not have a physical representation in the brain or any other organ that allows it to be diagnosed independently. Although there have been dozens of attempts to find such representations (they are called biomarkers), they have all failed. This does not mean they do not exist, but it is unlikely that all mental disorders will demonstrate an independent pathology. In short, although we can talk at length about the pharmacological properties of each drug with increasing degrees of accuracy, we come to a halt when we attempt to explain how they help in mental disorders.

PUTTING THE MODELS IN PERSPECTIVE: WHAT WE DEFINITELY KNOW

- *Mental illnesses are not diseases in the medical sense.* Every known medical disorder has a demonstrable body abnormality, whereas no mental disorder yet approaches this, despite many false claims over the years.
- *Even though as yet the exact nature of mental illness is unknown, it does not mean these conditions do not exist and can be discarded.* The nature of almost all physical disorders was completely unknown until the 20th century. Each mental disorder can be at least partly identified by diagnosis: the linking together of certain common features and/or behaviours so that together they can be viewed in the same way as medical diseases.
- *Diagnoses in psychiatry are not hard-wired like medical illnesses such as diabetes and heart failure, but neither are they useless when it comes to choosing treatments.* They are the current best guess of the nature of mental disorders and should be treated with respect but not slavish following. They can point towards successful treatment with drugs or psychological treatments.
- *Many old, now-discarded, drugs were basically stimulants or sedatives.* These include chloral hydrate and cocaine. But all currently prescribed drugs have a degree of specificity (i.e. their actions are linked to particular abnormalities via diagnosis) and so are chosen accordingly. This does not mean they are correcting a chemical imbalance any more than a good square meal corrects a dietary imbalance; it is just that the properties of the drug, its pharmacology, are relevant to the reversal of symptoms identified by the diagnosis.
- *The most successful drug treatment is one that relieves symptoms and improves function and, when considered to be no longer needed, can be withdrawn without any problems.* The proponents of the drug-centred model may have a valid point in predicting that withdrawal problems are natural consequences of stopping substances that 'produce global alterations to normal bodily processes, mental states and behaviour' (Moncrieff, 2020, p. 7). Drug specificity is only partial; we cannot pretend that other mental activities are entirely unaffected by them. But, as will become clear later in this book, 'withdrawal' is an elastic term that can be stretched in many different directions, and it should not always be linked to drugs themselves.
- *All drugs can be prescribed inappropriately and for excessively long periods.* The great increase in prescriptions of antidepressants without any reduction in suicide rates is often jumped on with alacrity by those who claim these drugs are useless at relieving depression. But would

they conclude the same about the massive increase in hip and knee replacements in recent years, a statistic that can be interpreted as a disgraceful epidemic of arthritis promoted by unscrupulous knife-happy orthopaedic surgeons who are in overdrive and desperate for custom? It is also worth emphasising that there are no treatments that have been shown unequivocally to reduce the suicide rate, so this particular comparison is of little value.

- *It is commonly asserted that as drugs are heavily promoted by Big Pharma (the collective name for both ethical and less-than-ethical drug companies), psychiatrists are duped, bribed and seduced into prescribing many more drugs than if they were sensible and judicious prescribers.* While this claim has some justification in some instances, much less so now than in the recent past, it is trotted out indiscriminately as a reason to abhor all drug treatment, and this is just cheap and shoddy logic.

BRIEF HISTORY OF DRUG TREATMENT IN PSYCHIATRY

It is always educational to examine the historical aspects of current behaviour and attitudes. Before the 19th century, almost all drug remedies were poisonous extracts of medicinal plants, and the only way they could be prevented from killing people was to boil, grill or denature them so that any benefit might occasionally be achieved in diluted form. For instance, the common foxglove, *Digitalis purpurea*, was shown by an astute physician, William Withering, to correct heart failure, and extracts from cinchona bark were found to treat malaria as they contained quinine. No such breakthroughs took place in the drug treatment of mental illness, and the only drug of note, laudanum, or opium, derived from the opium poppy, *Papaver somniferum*, spoiled its ability to sedate safely by being highly addictive. Barbiturates replaced opium but turned out to be almost as addictive.

Little of note was noted until 1950, when chlorpromazine, first introduced to lower blood pressure in patients undergoing operations, was found to have calming properties independent of general sedation. It was later used in the treatment of psychotic disorders, particularly schizophrenia, and in a range of trials shown to be effective in reducing delusions and hallucinations as well as having sedative value. Bearing in mind that at that time, all mental hospitals were bulging to overflowing with patients who were rarely receiving effective treatments, a new treatment that actually helped the features of severe mental illness was an absolute boon. Very soon afterwards, depression was next on the list to have effective drug treatment, initially with monoamine oxidase inhibitors (MAOIs) and later with imipramine, the first tricyclic antidepressant.

It is not surprising that such an abundance of fertility in the former psychiatric desert went to people's heads. So the 'psychopharmacological revolution' was born and the mental hospital population started declining from the mid-1950s onwards. There is some dispute about the reasons for this, as although the new drugs had a role, this was aided by the simultaneous growth of community psychiatry, helping to combat the debilitating effects of institutionalisation and promote reintegration into the community.

Dozens of new drugs were introduced in the 1960s and 1970s, but many of these were no more than replicas of existing drug groups, so the revolutionary zeal was flagging a little. It was not helped by the greater recognition of the adverse effects of many drugs, which had rarely been considered in the onward rush of enthusiasm for innovatory compounds. These included the development of abnormal movements of the mouth and limbs. This was termed tardive dyskinesia, and it often developed later in treatment with antipsychotic drugs such as chlorpromazine and trifluoperazine. It was then found that many anti-anxiety drugs (minor tranquillizers) were not fundamentally different from the barbiturates in creating a form of dependence not primarily associated with escalation of dosage but with unpleasant symptoms following withdrawal.

Pharmaceutical companies were highly influential in changing psychiatric practice in the latter years of the 20th century. They had many wares to promote and were very assiduous in courting psychiatrists to change their practice to the new drugs on offer, but this was deceptive, as by the 1980s, drug innovation was tailing off. However, the recognition of adverse effects with original antipsychotic drugs (Parkinsonism, sedation and tardive dyskinesia), tricyclic antidepressants (sedation and the anticholinergic effects of constipation, difficulty in micturition and dry mouth) and minor tranquillizers (dependence potential) led to a new approach. Drugs that were variants of old ones, not genuine novel drugs, were introduced and heavily promoted by the now highly profitable pharmaceutical industry, now called Big Pharma to show its gargantuan proportions. The two main classes were the selective serotonin reuptake inhibitors, commonly abbreviated to SSRIs, and the atypical antipsychotic or neuroleptic drugs.

These were promoted as safer alternatives to the 'failed' tricyclic antidepressants and old antipsychotics, not only more effective but much better tolerated, and led to a big increase in sales. But the claims were overstated. Clinical trials established that the new antidepressants did not have the unpleasant anticholinergic effects of the tricyclic compounds but had a host of new adverse effects including nausea, dizziness, insomnia and emotional numbness. Other trials showed no superiority of the atypical antipsychotic drugs over the old-fashioned compounds and although abnormal movement disorders were reduced, other new side effects, notably weight gain leading to type II diabetes, nausea and sleep disturbance, replaced them. In some patients, these were sufficiently severe to lead to a return to the original typical antipsychotic drugs.

In short, the present situation with drug therapy in psychiatry can perhaps best be summarised as 'steady as she goes'. Twelve years ago I suggested the psychopharmacological revolution was over as so many other non-drug treatments were competing for the same disorders (Tyrer, 2012). This is probably true at the time of writing, as there have been no major breakthroughs in drug treatment in the past 10 years, just a period of consolidation.

THE INTELLIGENT PRESCRIBER MODEL

So what model should the intelligent prescriber follow when deciding on drug therapy? I have previously described the model I have used for years in a book that was first published in 1989, *Models for Mental Disorder*, now in its sixth edition (Tyrer, 2022a). This makes it clear that mental illness cannot be subsumed within a single model that applies across all conditions. There are disease, behavioural, dynamic and social models at different stages of disorder, and the important task of the prescriber is to be aware of the severity and level of the disorder being treated. At the most severe level of disorder (e.g. impaired consciousness, severe behavioural disturbance in which mental capacity is grossly impaired), drug treatment is necessary simply to preserve life and to protect others. At this level of severity, it is appropriate to think of the disease model even though there is no physical representation of disease in the brain in most instances. At the opposite end of the spectrum, we have a group of conditions that could be regarded as normal variation rather than illness. These include mild personality problems, temporary changes in mood and behaviour, and what are called adjustment disorders, in which there is temporary disturbance occurring after environmental stress. Here the position of drug treatment is much less certain and requires much greater care.

At this level of disorder, it is absolutely necessary to bring the patient into the prescriber's confidence and, ideally, leave choice to the patient. It will be noted in the rest of this book that for these disorders, there is no clear evidence that drugs are superior to other forms of treatment and that much depends on the patient's choice. However, the choice has to be made in the light of knowledge. The prescriber needs to transfer this knowledge in advance of any choice being made. For many people this could be superseded by the common response, 'Do what you think is best, doctor?' But this is a cop out, and requires the response, 'It is not for me to decide what is best because in this subject there is no best and no worst choice. Whatever we decide, you are going to be the person taking, and living with, the treatment for as long as it lasts, so your views are much more important than mine'.

There is a great deal of concern with power in the therapeutic transactions of mental health professionals. This is relevant when patients are just given treatment without any proper explanation, but the intelligent prescriber should not be concerned about power in his or her relationships with patients. Why? Because the situations in which the patient has no say in treatment, as with severe mental disorder and lack of mental capacity, there is no alternative to the therapist controlling treatment and exercising power.

At the other end of the spectrum the threat of power disappears. The patient is given all the relevant information about the disorder and its treatment, and is free to choose drug or psychological treatment or to have any other intervention. The therapist may be asked, 'If you were me, doctor, what would you choose?' It's not an easy question to answer. It can be avoided by the response, 'I do not know you well enough to answer that question; I would probably choose xy treatment, but this may be quite inappropriate for you'.

CENTRAL MESSAGES OF CHAPTER 1

1. A single model to justify drug action in mental illness is not possible.

2. Joint agreement between patients and prescribers is best able to determine if a drug is of value without the need for models.

2

WHAT SHOULD PATIENTS KNOW ABOUT PSYCHOTROPIC DRUGS?

The times when patients took the advice of doctors without questions have long gone. The advent of the Internet, and the ubiquitous physician Dr Google, who knows everything and nothing and sometimes gets them mixed up, means that every utterance of a doctor can be questioned and checked and usually requires further amplification. Greater knowledge is always desirable, and more knowledge about the medications that enter their bodies can only be an asset. This is not to deny that ignorance may sometimes have its own advantages. Knowing a lot about one's own health is not always useful, especially if you are highly anxious and see a catastrophe around every corner. Such catastrophisers suffer from health anxiety, a growing problem that is probably being made worse by greater knowledge of illness, especially if you are learning from a non-scientific background (Hedman-Lagerlöf et al., 2019).

However, in general, if you are better informed, you are able to make better decisions about your health. I recently developed pains in my right leg after an operation on my left knee. I suspected this was because I was putting a strain on the good leg by making it do more work. But I could not understand why standard painkillers such as paracetamol had no effect on this pain. The answer came after an MRI showed very clearly that the nerves coming from the base of my spine were being nipped, so my spinal surgeon could make a diagnosis. The injury is called a radiculopathy, a form of sciatica, and was probably generated by putting too much strain on my right side and lower back. This type of pain is called neuropathic pain – pain generated by the nerves, not the muscles – and it does not respond to standard painkillers. It does respond to several psychotropic drugs, however,

DOI: 10.1201/9781032619019-3

and the oldest of these, amitriptyline, in a very small dose completely cleared up my symptoms after only 24 hours.

The other reason for describing this personal account is to point out that no mental health problem can be explained in a similar way. When Joanna Moncrieff writes that psychotropic drugs produce 'global alterations' to the body that are not fully understood, she is correct. The way in which a higher dose of amitriptyline relieves symptoms of depression cannot be explained in the same way that a lower dose relieves neuropathic pain. Why not? Because we cannot identify the exact site or nature of the change in depressive symptoms. We know it must be in the brain, and we know something about the neurotransmitters (molecules that act like a railway signal box in transmitting instructions to other cells), but this does not directly explain how depression is relieved. For many years, psychiatric researchers have been looking for biomarkers, identifiable biological changes that might indicate the fundamental building blocks of mental illness, but very little progress has been made to date.

HOW TO INTERPRET DRUG TREATMENT

As definitive answers cannot be given about the mechanism of psychotropic drug action, we have to be satisfied with partial explanations. Much of this comes from randomized controlled trials (see Chapter 5), the results of which tell the prescriber whether or not a drug is effective without explaining why or how efficacy is achieved. The trouble here is the already noted problem that such trials only show the findings of groups. I have previously rephrased a line from Tennyson, 'so careful of the group it seems, so careless of the single trial' to describe the neglect of unpredicted individual response to a drug (Tyrer, 2008).

Therefore, it is always wrong to make predictions of success or failure when a drug is prescribed. The unexpected positive response may be due to a placebo effect (see Chapter 11) or to other reasons not directly connected to pharmacology, but it can nonetheless be real. A patient must never ask the question, 'Can you guarantee this drug will relieve my symptoms?' as the intelligent prescriber will always respond 'No'.

KNOWING WHEN DRUGS ARE NO LONGER ACTIVE

Almost daily, it is possible to read in newspapers about unusual behaviour, usually involving violence in order to be newsworthy, in which drugs both illegal and legal are blamed for the consequences. It is here that it is useful to have some knowledge of how drugs act when they are in the body and how long they remain active for. Here is one example. Some years ago, I was asked to give an expert opinion in a legal case when a patient had claimed that his violent attack on another man was 'alien to his character' and had been caused by a drug he had taken 36 hours earlier. The drug he had taken was a benzodiazepine, which clears from the body within 10 hours. This drug had no active metabolites (i.e. other compounds altered in the body which had the same effects), so I was able to write a report saying that at the time of the assault, his behaviour was not affected by the alleged drug. His defence failed.

This was a simple case. Ones which are much more complex involve claims that after repeated drug administration, its effects both positive and negative, can persist for many years after stopping the drug. These claims are very difficult to evaluate. Several years after stopping a drug, there is no possibility that it is still hidden in the body somewhere, but it is plausible that the drug has created some changes in the receptor systems in the body that have made the body more sensitive to stressful input and therefore created the symptoms that are causing so much concern.

So if you have symptoms that you have never had before, how can you relate them to a drug you took many years ago? The celebrated Cambridge psychologist Frederic Bartlett coined the expression 'effort after meaning' (Bartlett, 1932) to describe the tendency for all people to reconstruct their memories to make them into a coherent story. The footballer remembers his first foray with a tennis ball in a school playground; the violinist her first hearing of Beethoven's violin concerto; and the celebrity chef his first visit to a busy kitchen in which, in spite of the bustle, the heat and the noise, the food sat resplendent in perfect order. These memories may be partly correct or so peripheral as to be fictitious, but what matters is that they make up a coherent story that sticks in the memory. Others that do not fit into the narrative, or completely contradict it, are conveniently forgotten. So unexpected symptoms cannot be allowed to be unexpected for long. They need to be woven into an explanation linked to the past.

Does this mean that those people who complain of symptoms arising many years after they stopped a drug are being fooled? No, there has to be some doubt here. It is well established that people who have lost a limb can still experience symptoms in the same limb even though it is no longer there. This phenomenon, known as phantom limb, is well described and is extremely common. Many explanations have been given for phantom limb experiences and most suggest that as the brain is 'hard-wired' into having messages from all parts of the body, it still expects to receive these when the limb is removed (De Ridder et al., 2014). Similarly, if you have had many years of unpleasant symptoms and these persist after drug treatment is stopped, this could be explained by the brain expecting symptoms even though the drug was stopped many years before.

In the next chapter, more is explained about the fate of drugs in the body.

CENTRAL MESSAGES OF CHAPTER 2

1.   The collective evidence of the value of a drug can be offset entirely in an individual case.

2.   Do not assume that new symptoms can be unequivocally ascribed to drug effects.

3

WHAT HAPPENS WHEN DRUGS ENTER THE BODY

Car drivers do not need to know exactly what goes on when air and fuel enter a carburettor, a spark flies and the engine starts, but they do need to have a rough idea what to do if the car fails to move. Similarly, it is helpful for a person taking a drug to know something about drugs when they enter the body. This chapter describes the basics of pharmacokinetics, which in simple language is the movement (kinetics) of drugs (pharma) in and out of the body.

A. HOW CAN DRUGS BE ADMINISTERED?

Drugs can be given in four different ways: directly into the body by injection into a vein, artery, muscle or skin; absorbed directly in the mouth; taken into the rectum or vagina in the form of pessaries or, most frequently, by being absorbed by the stomach and gut after swallowing. The most rapid effects are shown when the drug is given directly into the bloodstream through a vein, and this method is used by anaesthetists when they put people to sleep before an operation or for the rapid relief of intolerable pain.

B. WHAT HAPPENS TO DRUGS ONCE THEY ARE IN THE BODY?

Once drugs enter the body they are distributed around the different compartments, in the blood and plasma (the part of the blood containing cells and proteins), in the brain and other organs. Later, the drugs are eliminated, usually in the liver or kidneys. As all drugs that are absorbed through the stomach, gut or rectum pass through the liver, an organ

DOI: 10.1201/9781032619019-4

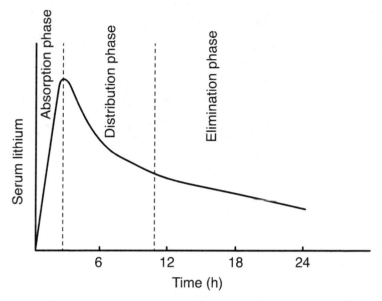

Figure 3.1   The absorption, distribution and elimination of lithium.

that also breaks down drugs, the amount detected in the body may be a great deal less than the dosage given. The pathway of one of the simplest of psychiatric drugs, lithium, is shown in Figure 3.1. Most other drugs follow a similar pathway which varies from drug to drug. The speed at which drugs pass into the brain is also variable, some do not get into the brain at all while others pass through the 'blood-brain barrier', as it is called, with ease.

C. WHAT HAPPENS TO DRUGS WHEN GIVEN REPEATEDLY?

When a drug is given frequently, the blood levels will increase if the frequency of administration exceeds the speed of elimination. With all drugs, there is a therapeutic range within which positive effects are shown, a sub-therapeutic one when the drug is not taken in sufficient dosage to produce benefit and a toxic range at which the drug could produce harmful effects (Figure 3.2)

The term 'therapeutic index' is used to describe the ratio of the toxic to the therapeutic dose. For some drugs (e.g. benzodiazepines), this is very high (i.e. the drug is safe even in high dosage), but for others it is low (e.g. lithium has a therapeutic index of just over 2).

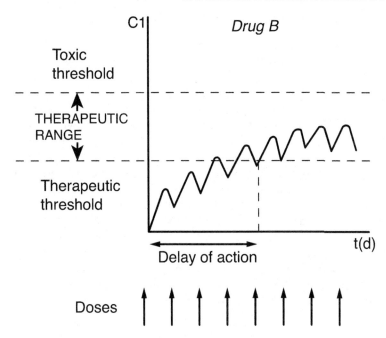

Figure 3.2 The accumulation of drug effects after repeated administration in a drug with an intermediate or long half-life.

D. AT WHAT POINT IS THE BENEFIT OF A DRUG SHOWN?

For some drugs (e.g. most of the tranquillizer group), the benefit is shown when the blood level reaches the therapeutic zone (as in Figure 3.2), but for many others, there is a delay of up to several weeks. It is not fully understood why there is this delay, and why it should take only a short time in some people and a much longer time in others. The reason for this is that receptors in the brain have to go through a period of adjustment or retuning before the new drug can show its value.

The main problem in practice is that adverse effects do not show the courtesy of a delay in their effects. These are usually shown immediately after a drug is taken and are often worse at first rather than later. This is one of the important reasons why patients should be clear about all the effects of psychotropic drugs before starting therapy.

E. HOW DO DRUGS LEAVE THE BODY?

Drugs lose their effects in the body in two ways. The first is through metabolism, the alteration of drugs by enzymes in the body. Enzymes are proteins that either break down drugs to simpler forms or convert them to other compounds that can have the same properties as the original drugs. Thus, for example, enzymes convert the common tranquilliser, diazepam, to a similar substance, desmethyldiazepam, which has the same properties as diazepam.

The second method is that they are ejected from the body, first being broken down (metabolized) to inactive compounds and then being eliminated via the kidneys and leave the body in the urine, or broken down in the liver. If patients have the function of their livers or kidneys impaired for any reason, drugs may accumulate to toxic levels; certain drugs then have to be avoided, and when prescribed need lower doses.

The other important property all need to know about a drug is its half-life in the body. That is the amount of time it takes for half of the drug in the body to be lost, either through metabolism or excretion. The half-life of a drug can vary from less than an hour to many weeks, and this has an important bearing on the effects of the drug. The half-life of the active metabolites is also important. The half-life of desmethyldiazepam is 96 hours, more than twice the half-life of its parent, diazepam, and as desmethyldiazepam is also metabolized to another active drug, oxazepam (half-life 8 hours), it is easy to see how drugs can accumulate in the body after frequent dosage.

F. THE IMPORTANCE OF PHARMACOKINETICS

It is not necessary for the average prescriber or patient to know a great deal about the pharmacokinetics of a drug, but I have described the basic elements. In practice, it is the effects a person notices about the drug in the body, its pharmacodynamics, that are more important, and on their own, pharmacokinetics has a relatively small part to play. A drug which shows blood levels to be in the normal range may still have toxic levels in the brain and elsewhere. The elderly, who are less able to metabolize and eliminate drugs from the body, may also show toxic effects when blood levels are within the normal range.

But it is useful to know something about the pharmacokinetics of drugs when deciding on how frequently they should be taken, so in other parts of this book, the half-life and metabolites may be mentioned when they are relevant, particularly when drug combinations are being considered and withdrawal problems described.

CENTRAL MESSAGES OF CHAPTER 3

1. All patients who take psychotropic drugs should know at least something about what happens when they enter the body (their pharmacokinetics).

2. Knowing when a drug is likely to start showing both its beneficial and adverse effects can be helped by understanding pharmacokinetics.

4

ESSENTIAL ELEMENTS TO UNDERSTAND IN PRESCRIBING

Do drugs help people with mental illness? The answer is a qualified 'yes', but it is only really true if both patient and prescriber are properly informed. 'Take these tablets and you will be better in four weeks' is not an informed statement. The prescription of a drug has to follow the eight steps of prescribing that also help to answer the four key questions that patients often ask at the same time:

1. **C**haracteristics and name of the drug prescribed
2. **H**elp expected from prescription
3. **A**dvantages and disadvantages in comparison to other therapies
4. **I**njury – risk of serious harm from the drug
5. **N**umber to be prescribed and in what frequency
6. **S**peed of action
7. **A**dverse effects
8. **W**ithdrawal problems that should be known before first prescription

The key questions that patients need to ask can be represented by the acronym WIDE:

- **W**hat is the drug?
- **I**s it safe and effective?
- **D**oes it have side effects, or problems with other drugs or alcohol?
- **E**xactly when do I expect benefits and how long will I need the drug for?

I note that the eight elements also spell the acronym CHAINSAW, which is a useful implement for cutting down unnecessary verbiage. The questions asked in WIDE will also be answered in simple language. The details of the individual drugs and their usage comes in the following chapter.

DOI: 10.1201/9781032619019-5

CHARACTERISTICS OF THE DRUG

As noted earlier, a drug can be given directly into the tissues of the body by an injection, usually just below the skin (subcutaneous) or into a muscle on the arm or leg (intramuscular), by mouth, where some can be absorbed under the tongue (sublingual), in the nose (intra-nasal) or, much more commonly, in the stomach and small intestine. Almost all common prescriptions are given in pill form or as a solution. If given as a pill or capsule, this form of administration is usually not stated, but if the patient has problems swallowing pills, this ought to be made clear at this point in the consultation.

Understanding the name of the drug can be a problem. Most drugs are advertised under the preferred name of the manufacturer, commonly called a trade name that indicates the ownership of the drug. New drugs are patented, and for the 20 years after its invention, no other manufacturer is allowed to create that drug. However, the patent is normally not granted for several years after invention, and in practice, exclusive marketing of the drug lasts for about 10 years. After this time, other manufacturers often create the drug, usually in different forms and dosage, and provide another trade name.

In this book, all drugs are described by their *approved* names, which do not change from country to country and are independent of the manufacturing source. On every prescription, in addition to the trade name often emblazoned on the front of the packet, in smaller letters you will see the approved name of the drug. The pharmacist will also affix a label giving the approved name in case it is forgotten by the manufacturer.

HELP EXPECTED

The prescriber should always indicate the type of help expected from the drug prescribed, but when giving a psychotropic drug, do not expect the word 'cure' or doubt it if it happens to be uttered. Having absolute confidence in the success of treatment is not the stuff of mental illness. For many conditions such as dementia and incurable cancer, the most that can be offered is a delay in the progression of the illness. For other conditions such as depression and psychosis of all types, drugs may relieve symptoms and improve behaviour, but no guarantee can be made about the length of time that treatment will be needed. For brief episodes of distress, often called adjustment reactions, more confidence can be expressed: 'You have a condition which is very likely to get completely better. I am going to prescribe a drug that I think will take away your symptoms and which will need to be taken for only a few weeks' is a correct response here.

You will note that correct advice requires a good knowledge of the condition being treated. No drug should be given for symptoms in a diagnostic vacuum.

INJURY AND HAZARDS

All drugs have side effects, but it would be wrong to regard these as trumping all the beneficial ones. Most prescriptions, at least those given for the first time, have an accompanying leaflet giving a list of all the possible adverse effects. You should not read this if you are in a nervous or contrary mood, because if you do, you will be inclined not to take a single dose. All manufacturers have to give a list of adverse effects, and although this is prudent, it is important to have some idea of how common each of them is.

Table 4.1 lists all the side effects noticed during a drug trial lasting 12 months, offering a better perspective on the side effects of drugs. You might think that this list of problems should make both prescriber and patient think again before giving a prescription for this drug, but some of the effects described are probably not related to the drug in any way.

What is this drug behind these effects? Not the experimental drug, lamotrigine, but the placebo, a dummy pill taken in order to compare its effects with an active drug. Many of these symptoms or problems appeared during the year even though in theory, a placebo should have no effects. The placebo group actually had 40 more adverse events in this year than the active drug group, so it is wise not to automatically attribute a list of adverse events to the active drug concerned.

The other difficulty is the interpretation of very rare events after taking the drug, such as death. It is often extremely difficult to decide exactly what is the cause of death. For instance, if it is found that there was only one death among 200 patients taking a drug for five years (i.e. 100 years of drug exposure), that death is highly unlikely to be due to the drug. But if there are five deaths, and the circumstances are all very similar (e.g. a heart attack), then there may be an association. This is one of the reasons why those with heart disease receive special warnings in the side effect leaflets.

The common side effects of drugs, as opposed to the uncommon ones that can be shown at any time, are usually shown early in treatment and tend to decrease over time. But there is great variation here and sometimes an effect that seems tolerable at first, for example, dizziness, can become more serious with repeated dosage and lead to the patient stopping the drug.

Table 4.1 Adverse Events in 139 Patients Taking Part in a Randomized Trial Lasting 52 Weeks

Total number of adverse events	285
Total number of participants with at least one adverse event	93
Total number of adverse events by system organ class:	
1. Blood and lymphatic system disorders	3
2. Cardiac disorders	1
3. Endocrine disorders	1
4. Eye disorders	6
5. Gastrointestinal disorders	55
6. General disorders and administration site conditions	14
7. Hepatobiliary disorders	0
8. Immune system disorders	1
9. Infections and infestations	38
10. Injury, poisoning and procedural complications	39
11. Investigation	3
12. Metabolism and nutrition disorders	1
13. Musculoskeletal and connective tissue disorders	7
14. Pregnancy, puerperium and perinatal conditions	2
15. Psychiatric disorders	40
16. Renal and urinary disorders	0
17. Reproductive system and breast disorders	1
18. Respiratory, thoracic and mediastinal disorders	9
19. Skin and subcutaneous tissue disorders	31
20. Social circumstances	1
21. Surgical and medical	
22. Procedures	1

Source: Data extracted from Crawford et al. (2018), (Table 11) with permission from the authors and Health Technology Assessment.

NUMBER OF TABLETS AND FREQUENCY

A new prescription of a psychotropic drug is usually for a short time only, up to three weeks. If the drug is entirely new to the patient, a low dose may be recommended at first because of the possibility of side effects. This explains the wide variety in drug dosage described in Chapter 13. It is wise to start low, but a nervous patient may be wary of raising the dose and stay on this low dose for too long. All drugs have a therapeutic range, a dosage developed from experience which needs to be attained before it is effective. If the patient never takes a dosage high enough to reach the therapeutic range, it may be abandoned prematurely as ineffective.

Many prescriptions indicate when the tablets should be taken, including the times of day and whether before or after meals. These instructions need not always be followed to the letter: if a pill's prescription says 'every 6 hours', it does not mean the person has to be a slave to the message and set an alarm to be woken in the night to keep to the exact times. The instructions may sometimes need to be over-ruled. For example, many of the newer antidepressant drugs (SSRIs) are alerting ones and so are better taken in the morning. But a minority of patients find they are sedating, and under these circumstances, the drugs are better taken in the evening, often close to bedtime.

Repeat prescriptions need not follow the first in indicating dosage. If the patient makes it clear at the second appointment that a different method of dosage has been followed and is seen as better, then even if the manufacturer's recommendations are clearly contradictive, the patient's views will often win the day. Any patient who is unhappy with a drug, for any reason, is more likely to stop taking it, and this is in nobody's interest.

SPEED OF ACTION

A patient wanting relief from unpleasant symptoms needs to know the time course of the drug's actions in the body. If the symptoms are in the anxiety dimension, many drugs can at least partially relieve these symptoms within 30 minutes. The standard anti-anxiety drugs such as benzodiazepines and antihistamines are absorbed quickly and exert their sedative effects rapidly. If no change is noticed within an hour or so of taking the drug, this may be because the symptoms are so intense that the benefit is not shown.

Prescriptions often anticipate this with instructions such as 'take up to four times a day'. This allows the option of taking up to four tablets within the space of a few hours. Such a prescription is not an encouragement to overdose but allows the value of the drug to be matched to the intensity of symptoms. The word 'titrate' is often used here. This is a word coming from chemistry that describes the gradual increase of a substance being added to another until the two substances combine in an expected reaction, and titrating the dose of an anti-anxiety drug until it induces calm is similar. But there is a danger here; the total daily dose should not be exceeded because it would then come into the realm of overdosage and potential danger. Excessive sedation can slow down major centres in the brain and lead to respiratory or cardiac collapse.

ADVERSE EFFECTS

The most common adverse (side) effects of psychotropic drugs are gastrointestinal (stomach and gut upsets), including nausea, stomach pains and constipation or diarrhoea; sedation (feeling drowsy or sleepy); dizziness or feeling light-headed; dry mouth, poor concentration and irritability or agitation. These are not only very common but also non-specific in that they do not necessarily follow from the nature of the drug being prescribed. In case of doubt, look at Table 4.1 again – all these symptoms were found with placebo tablets.

More importantly, if other adverse effects are described in the drug information packages, particularly those referring to cardiac, kidney, liver or respiratory disease, you may be advised not to take the drug or, if it is permitted, to take it in a much lower dose. If the main breakdown (metabolism) is in the liver or kidney and you have impaired function in these organs, the drug may accumulate to toxic levels.

Most adverse effects are found early in treatment, and this is the main reason prescribers often suggest starting treatment at a low level before increasing to the recommended dose. Normally, by the time the first prescription is finished, the adverse effects will have either disappeared or lessened. If they still constitute a problem, the drug may have to be changed. Manufacturers are often criticized for having too many drugs with similar treatment profiles available for prescription – they are dubbed 'me-too' drugs – but if they are similar in effect but have different adverse effects, they can be a boon to patients who cannot tolerate the first drug prescribed.

My final word in this section is to those who are excessively concerned about their health and fear disease around every corner. These people are said to have health anxiety, and they take a great deal of notice of drug information leaflets, which are almost always very accurate but also consult that well-known expert, Dr Google on the Internet, before they take a prescribed drug. Dr Google may be right, he may be wrong, but he often exaggerates dangers and has the habit of implying, if not always directly stating, that rare and potentially fatal consequences of taking a drug have been reported. As noted in the section on injury, it is often very difficult to be certain if a rare adverse effect is caused by a drug. When Dr Google makes a statement such as 'one in 200,000 people may get this serious reaction', the patient with health anxiety is prone to saying 'never mind the 200,000, I know I am the one who will get this awful reaction'. So it is wise for the health anxious person to stick to the real experts when looking for evidence.

WITHDRAWAL PROBLEMS

This is currently the most contentious part of the prescribing process. Because of all the attention given to withdrawal difficulties in the media, both mainstream and social media, it is perfectly proper for a patient to ask a doctor when receiving the first prescription of a drug, 'Will I have problems in stopping the drug when it is no longer needed?' Although this is a fair question, it cannot always be answered honestly, for reasons that become apparent in the rest of this book. Almost all medications, including placebo, can lead to withdrawal problems, so if the doctor replies 'absolutely not' to the patient's question posed, he or she is either being extremely rash or he knows the patient very well indeed. Why should knowing the patient well be of such value? By the time you get to the end of this book, you will have the answer.

If the doctor or other prescriber feels concerned about the possibility of withdrawal problems, a drug with very low dependence potential (see Chapter 7) may be prescribed, even if it not the best drug for the condition. This has to be explained in honesty and good faith: 'I am worried that you may have problems in withdrawing from the drugs that might be most effective in treating your condition, but because you and I are both a little concerned about you getting dependent I am going to prescribe a different drug. This might be a little less effective, but it will be much easier to stop'.

It is much better if this question is addressed as early as possible in treatment. The time of first prescription is ideal. Of course, there are many patients who never contemplate any problems of withdrawal and wonder why the subject is addressed at all, but it is wise for the prescriber to mention withdrawal problems early in the consultation process. If it is not mentioned and as a patient you are concerned, please bring the question up before you leave with your prescription. To summarize the absolute essentials to satisfy patients at their consultations with prescribers, preferably at the first meeting, I return to WIDE.

WHAT IS THE DRUG?

Although this is almost certainly mentioned by the prescriber, it is not often explained in full. This can hardly be expected in an average consultation lasting around six minutes, but it is reasonable to ask what type of drug it is and why it has been chosen. In the last chapter of this book, I have listed all the approved names of drugs that are marketed in most countries.

IS IT SAFE?

Dangerous drugs are not available for general prescription, so the answer to this question will almost always be positive, but this is also the time to ask about difficulties in stopping the drug. It will be difficult to give a straight answer to this question for reasons related to withdrawal discussed elsewhere in this book. But a rough reply such as 'I only expect you to need one or, at the most, two prescriptions, so we should not have problems stopping it' is reasonably accurate and can be reassuring. Because of the dangers of drug and alcohol interactions you as a patient may also be asked about your consumption of alcohol and other drugs, both legal and illegal. If you are not able to reply honestly, problems could arise later, and you may not be taking a safe combination of drugs.

DOES IT HAVE SIDE EFFECTS?

If the prescriber, be it doctor, nurse or psychologist, has experience with the drug concerned, this will be a great help in answering this question. The answer can then be made from knowledge of other patients' feedback, and this is usually reassuring. If you have a particular side effect in mind, this is the time to raise it.

EXACT TIME OF BENEFIT AND DURATION OF EFFECTS

It is very common for all prescribers to give some idea of the speed of action of any psychotropic drug when first given. The main difficulty is separating the times of initial effects such as sedation from the underlying reason for prescribing the drug. In the case of longer-term disorders such as bipolar disorder or psychoses such as schizophrenia. it may be many weeks or months before the positive effects are known, especially when the drug is being prescribed as a maintenance drug to prevent relapse. It may seem obvious, but more complex explanations of benefit must be made before patients leave with their prescriptions.

CENTRAL MESSAGES FROM CHAPTER 4

1. When patients leave a clinic after a first prescription, they should know what is being prescribed, why and how it will help and any problems to be expected along the way.

2. Adverse events and their time course should be pointed out but not exaggerated.

5

DIAGNOSIS AND DRUG INDICATIONS

Psychotropic drugs are not prescribed as uppers or downers, as panaceas for all types of mental illness or as convenient fodder for drug companies fleecing an unsuspecting public. The drug–centred model of mental illness described in Chapter 1 gives the wrong impression that the complexities of mental illness have a common base, that all is stirred up by giving drugs that we know little about apart from the division between sedation and stimulation. It also adds there is not much difference between different drugs, and we wrongly attribute mechanisms of action that have no basis in fact. This model is based on half-truths – the absence of biomarkers for mental illness, the poor quality of drug mechanisms that always seem to follow clinical evidence instead of informing it and the fads of prescribing unnecessarily – and can be seductive.

But there is science behind the prescription of these drugs, and it is good science at least in part, capable of being tested and disproved and harnessed in a form that makes prescription logical and more effective. Part of this better use of drugs depends on diagnosis. Although the absence of bodily indicators of mental illness, apart from some exceptions such as dementia, makes psychiatric diagnosis more suspect than medical diagnosis, it does not make it invalid. People can deny depression exists as there is no part of the nervous or immune system that can be identified as abnormal, but it does not make depression a non-disease. You cannot invalidate a deeply held feeling shared by millions of others by saying it cannot exist as we cannot find it in the brain. Depression is as real as a brain tumour; it is just that we cannot yet find it (even though Professor Bullmore in Cambridge claims it is all due to inflammation [Bullmore, 2020]).

DOI: 10.1201/9781032619019-6

Therefore, when choosing to give a psychiatric drug, we need to know something about the patterns of response. Some people seem to get completely better, others a little better and some hardly at all. The whole population cannot just be divided up in this way. If we had no means of differentiating responders and non-responders, prescription would become a total lottery.

This is where psychiatric diagnosis comes in. Compared with medical diagnosis, where the organs that are diseased can be identified and studied in the most minute detail, psychiatric diagnosis is confined to a low division in the league, the equivalent of Third Division North in the English football league compared with the big players of heart, liver, brain and kidney disease in the Premier League. But in the football league clubs can get promoted or relegated; those in the psychiatric Third Division are destined to stay permanently near the bottom until what others call 'real disease' can be found.

But this does not mean psychiatric diagnosis is worthless. Many supporters of Third Division North clubs will confirm they often see good football. It is just we cannot have the same degree of confidence in our team labels as they can in the big leagues, and often we have to abandon diagnoses and replace them with others (in football this is called 'going into administration').

So both patients and prescribers need to be aware when they talk about drugs for certain psychiatric diagnoses that they are not on entirely firm territory. What they do get angry about are claims that they are just following a false trail led by drug companies and that diagnosis does not properly exist. What follows in this chapter is a set of linkages between drug prescription and diagnosis that is very much better than having no diagnostic system at all. Each section is headed by one of the main diagnostic groups used in the latest world classification of mental disorders, ICD-11. (This was introduced in January 2022 but has not yet been implemented in some countries, but it is the up-to-date classification.)

EFFECTIVENESS

In describing each of the drugs and drug groups, I am only including those that have been confirmed as being effective from evidence of randomized controlled trials. There are mixed views about randomized trials, but it is rightly concluded that the best evidence of the effectiveness of any drug treatment comes from well-designed studies in which patients are chosen at random to receive either the drug under investigation or an inert placebo and assessments of outcome made at fixed intervals afterwards. If this is done properly, the natural bias that people have of favouring the active drug is removed.

What is important in such trials is to have a primary outcome decided in advance. This may not seem important, but if you have many different outcome measurements and one turns out to show a significant difference, it could be a chance finding. There is also an unfortunate tendency for trials hosted by drug companies to have more positive results than those carried out by independent investigators. This is partly because the trials showing negative results often remain unpublished and also because trials with multiple outcomes with many different measured time points are more likely to find a positive somewhere and this is then given a false priority. There is more rigour needed in trials today than in the past (see a fictional account based on fact in an illuminating book [Eagles, 2023]), but in general, bodies evaluating the efficacy of drugs such as the National Institute of Health and Care Excellence (NICE) feel much more confident about efficacy when they have positive results from trials that have independent oversight.

However, there is one important aspect of randomized controlled trials that can properly be interpreted as a criticism. These trials compare the results of groups of patients and the data for individual patients are subsumed, and sometimes lost, within the groups. A trial may show no benefit for a drug when groups are compared, but hidden within the groups, there may be individuals who responded to the drug but are not recognised in the data unless the trials are very large indeed. Small trials often show no differences between drug and placebo even though important differences may be present. This is because the numbers are said to lack power; if the same results were found with twice the numbers enroled, the differences would then often show as significant.

These points become important when prescribers are using drugs that are second- or third-line options (often because the first-line one has failed) and there are few data available on the new drug. It in these cases that the past experience the prescriber has with the drug is so important. It is also important to listen carefully to patients when they insist a drug that is not normally prescribed for their condition has helped them enormously. The response may show that the person is unusual but the benefit is nonetheless real; the hidden responder in a controlled trial should not be universally suppressed.

PSYCHOSIS AND DRUG TREATMENT

This group includes the conditions that have previously been diagnosed as schizophrenia, but this is now recognised to be too specific. Instead, psychosis in ICD-11 includes schizophrenia and many related syndromes, including schizoaffective and delusional disorder, all of which can be described as primary psychotic disorders (Gaebel & Salveridou-Hof, 2023).

One of the reasons for the change in diagnosis is to give more weight to acute presentations of these conditions. 'Acute and transient psychotic disorders', as they are called, only last for a few days and very rarely beyond three months. These conditions look like the standard features of schizophrenia as they have the same symptoms – hallucinations, disorganized thinking, notions of the mind or body being controlled – but they come out of the blue, often at times of considerable stress. The importance of this distinction is that the standard medication for schizophrenia, antipsychotic drugs that I describe shortly, are only likely to be needed for a short time in these conditions. In most cases, admission to hospital is needed, and it is clear by the time of discharge that the condition is an acute one, but it is most important that recommendations for both continuing and stopping drug treatment are followed.

There is another diagnosis in the psychotic group that was in the past closely linked to schizophrenia called delusional disorder. This is not like an acute psychotic episode as symptoms like hallucinations and disorganized thinking are not present, and unlike acute episodes, the symptoms tend to persist, often for years. This disorder has not been studied as carefully as some others, but in general, drug treatment has not been as successful as in other psychoses, even though it is widely used (Lähteenvuo et al., 2021).

The main drugs used for treating psychosis are the antipsychotic drugs. This is an obvious collective description, but it can be confusing as these drugs are now used in a range of conditions. A common error is to assume that the prescription of an antipsychotic drug automatically means the sufferer has an illness in the schizophrenia group. These drugs now have much wider use in mood disorders and anxiety disorders (in lower dosages).

There are many antipsychotic drugs (each is listed in Chapter 13), but they can be usefully divided into two groups, typical and atypical. The typical group includes most of the early drugs introduced into psychiatry – chlorpromazine, trifluoperazine, flupenthixol, haloperidol and prochlorperazine. These were found early to produce movement disorders (extrapyramidal side effects), mainly akathisia, a subjective feeling of restlessness, particularly affecting the legs; parkinsonism (slowing of movement, tremor (shaking) and muscle rigidity) and, less commonly, acute dystonias, when many muscles go into spasm. These adverse effects can be corrected to a large extent with anticholinergic drugs. A more resistant adverse effect is tardive dyskinesia, the later development of abnormal writhing movements of the face, hands and body. This tends to occur after several years of treatment and is generally resistant to medication.

These adverse effects are unpleasant and very bothersome for most people, so it is not surprising that there was a search for other drugs of similar efficacy with fewer adverse consequences. The atypical antipsychotic drugs have similar efficacy to their typical equivalents (Lieberman et al., 2005; Jones et al., 2006), but although they are less liable to abnormal movement problems, these still occur; the drugs also have the additional negative effects of weight gain, often leading to Type 2 diabetes mellitus (i.e. diabetes requiring treatment but rarely insulin), heart problems and sexual problems. Some of these have been less marked as newer drugs have been introduced, particularly amisulpiride, aripiprazole and risperidone. Olanzapine has sedative properties but is very prone to causing weight gain.

The antipsychotic drug that stands on its own in clozapine. It has different pharmacological properties than the other antipsychotic drugs, it was the first atypical antipsychotic and it is generally more effective than all others (Lewis et al., 2006), so it is often used when other drugs have failed (Kane et al., 1988; Chakos et al., 2001). But it has serious adverse effects, the most important being the loss of important blood cells (agranulocytosis) so that people are more prone to infection; this occurs in one in 100 of all patients treated. As a consequence, in most countries, regular blood tests to check on blood counts are an essential part of the treatment programme. Other side effects include inflammation of the heart (myocarditis), a fall in blood pressure (hypotension), sedation and excessive production of saliva in the mouth (an unusual condition called sialorrhoea). With this panoply of adverse effects, it takes a lot of debate before it is recommended that a patient take clozapine after failing to respond to other drugs.

Not all antipsychotic drugs are prone to extrapyramidal side effects. Many of the atypical group, including clozapine, quetiapine, aripiprazole, olanzapine, risperidone and several others are relatively free of these effects, so their prescription has taken over from the older drugs. The very unpleasant symptoms of movement disorder usually disappear over time if the antipsychotic drug is stopped. For acute symptoms, the drugs amantadine (a common treatment for Parkinson's disease itself), orphenadrine, procyclidine and benztropine will offset their emergence and are sometimes prescribed automatically. This anticipation of symptoms is called prophylaxis and is reasonable when a large dose of a typical antipsychotic is used, but it is not appropriate to add the antiparkisonian drug automatically.

Many antipsychotic drugs interfere with sexual function greatly and this also creates considerable distress. Very few of the drugs are completely free of this adverse effect.

It will not surprise many that a large number of patients do not relish taking these drugs and wish to stop them entirely. To aid adherence to the drug, many antipsychotic drugs are given by long-acting injections into the muscles of the shoulder or the buttock. These include slow-release preparations of flupenthixol, zuclopenthixol, olanzapine, risperidone and paliperidone in a form or substance (e.g. oil) that allows the drug to gradually enter the rest of the body.

What is the position of the patient when it comes to prescribing in psychoses? It is certainly not one of equal partnership. A large amount of treatment administration, at least initially, is by coercion, frequently by a section of the Mental Health Act, and long-term treatment is similarly coercive by instruments such as Community Treatment Orders. Patients can argue that they should have much more say in the treatment of their psychoses, and sometimes they are right. If I were a patient and was convinced that my psychosis was not a persistent illness but a brief recurring episodic one, I would move mountains to convince my doctors that continuous treatment was unnecessary.

One of my own patients, Anthea (she later changed her name), did just that. After spending several months in mental hospitals over a 17-year period, she convinced me after weeks of arguing that her psychosis was episodic, not continuous. I first tried to persuade her that the explanation of her symptoms may be true and that the best way of shortening her illness episodes was to take antipsychotic drugs as soon as she felt a relapse was imminent. But she would not have it. 'These drugs mess up my endocrine system – they are just poisonous'.

I acceded to her request to make her case in front of an audience of psychiatrists in training. 'Surely you must agree', one of them gently argued, 'that if you took the drugs when you were ill, you would have a much shorter period of your psychosis and might even avoid coming into hospital?' But she would not have it, and her reply was direct and forceful. 'Before you say that again, you must take all the drugs that I have been on and then let me know if you still believe it.' She won the day, and many in the audience were in sympathy.

In the end, the agreement we made was that when she had episodes of psychosis, she would confine herself to her flat, have no contact with anyone and live like a hermit until the episode was over. This worked. She continued to have short episodes annually but only had two short admissions in the subsequent 10 years. She wrote me a letter subsequently, using not quite the language I would have chosen, but which expresses her sentiments very well:

> *I am glad you have taken the freedom to treat patients according to your integrity and not by the book, so that you are an enlightened psychiatrist who makes his patients feel much better and not a psychopath who uses the system to vindicate his blind dogma of academic learning that inflicts so much helpless suffering in the name of medicine.*

(Tyrer, 2000, p. 255)

I am not suggesting that all patients with a psychotic illness can be as successful as Anthea in avoiding medication as her illness was an unusual one. But more notice should be given to the feedback given by patients who are keen on reducing or stopping their drugs. For those who develop a schizophrenia-like psychotic illness at an early age, particularly if it develops slowly, antipsychotic drugs may need to be given regularly over a long period. Those who stop, even if it is after many years of treatment, are much more likely to relapse than those who stay on the drugs (Tilhonen et al., 2018). The consequences of relapse may be severe; a very eloquent example of a murder following such a relapse is in a published report of an enquiry, *The Falling Shadow*, that can be read online (Blom-Cooper et al., 1995).

Patients at the other end of the psychosis spectrum may either not need the medications at all or have them for short periods only. This background emphasises the importance of correct diagnosis at the beginning of a psychotic illness. Many authorities feel that gains in outcome can be made by early intervention in psychotic illness so that the duration of illness is shorter and allegedly creates less permanent damage. But Joanna Moncrieff has rightly pointed out that 'people who develop psychosis gradually tend to come forward for treatment later in the course of their psychosis' (Moncrieff, 2020, p. 70), so the populations are not the same.

One of the dangers of early diagnosis in psychosis is that it may be wrong. This could lead to a lifetime of drug treatment, with all its adverse effects, which would be a pernicious consequence of error. In deciding whether a trial without drugs is justified, the history of the development of the psychosis is very important. When it has appeared suddenly, in the context of drug misuse, and has atypical features, there is a much better chance of full recovery when drug therapy is withdrawn.

Whenever drugs cause problems in treating mental illness, it is natural to look for alternatives, but these are not that encouraging for psychosis. Although psychological treatments such as cognitive behaviour therapy (CBT) have been used in the treatment of schizophrenia for many years (Kingdon & Turkington, 1994), they are of only limited value in the acute phases of the condition, and their value is mainly in the treatment of persistent symptoms and what are often called the 'negative symptoms' such as apathy, lack of motivation, reduced social involvement and depressive lack of interest (Sensky et al., 2000; Morrison et al., 2019). There is no proven psychological treatment for the acute positive symptoms of schizophrenia despite clarion calls for someone, somewhere, to provide one.

DEPRESSIVE DISORDERS

Depressive disorders cover a wide range of conditions, ranging from depressive stupor at one extreme, when the mind and body are slowed down to virtually zero, and mild depression at the other extreme, when people feel under par but are still able to carry out all their activities.

The symptoms of depression are very well known: low mood, pessimistic outlook on life, feeling that life is not worth living, lack of energy and interest, sleep disturbance with difficulty getting off to sleep and frequent waking in the night, loss of appetite followed by loss of weight, and a slowing down of all activities. In very severe depression, the sufferer may become mute and stuporose (not moving and being unresponsive) and develop delusions such as believing their bodies no longer exist (Cotard's syndrome).

For severe depression, there is really no alternative to drug therapy, or if very severe, electroconvulsive therapy, although this is becoming much less frequent as antidepressant drugs have improved. Very recently, a new set of drugs derived from ketamine, an anaesthetic and painkiller first used in the 1960s, has been shown to have antidepressant properties (Hashimoto, 2019). One of these derivatives, esketamine, has now been approved for the treatment of depression under specialist supervision, and it is given by an intranasal spray in a complex sequence (see list of drugs in Chapter 13). Treatment should be continued for at least six months after depressive symptoms improve. One always has to be cautious in assessing the initial effects of a new drugs, but the evidence to date is that this drug represents a real advance (Popova et al., 2020; Singh et al., 2020a). But, and it is a very big but, we need to find out all the possible adverse effects before we can recommend its widespread use.

It is often not necessary to treat depression with drugs; for a wide range of depression severity, psychological treatments, mainly talking therapies such as CBT are just as effective. However, these equal benefits that are sometimes superior at low levels of depression do not extend

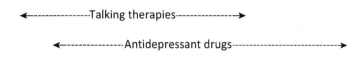

Figure 5.1 Choice of treatment in depressive disorders.

to severe depression (Figure 5.1). This is very important when it comes to choice of treatment. When Joanna Moncrieff writes, 'Combining data from all available trials, both published and unpublished, reveals that antidepressants have larger effects than placebo but the difference is vanishingly small' (Moncrieff, 2020, p. 79), she is bending the truth a little. For unequivocal moderate and severe depression, antidepressants are effective in relieving symptoms.

Antidepressant drugs are also divided into groups, the names of which have changed over time. The original antidepressants were named by their chemical structure, the tricyclic antidepressants, first introduced in the form of imipramine in 1953. Just previously, another group, the MAOIs, named after their pharmacological properties, had been introduced, but these are rarely used today, mainly because of concern over the danger of interaction with certain foods containing tyramine, an amine that raises the blood pressure. But many feel they still have a place in treatment when other antidepressants have failed.

TRICYCLIC ANTIDEPRESSANTS

Tricyclic antidepressants have common side effects, mostly anticholinergic effects (blocking the effects of an important brain substance, choline) that have reduced their general use. These include sedation, constipation, dry mouth, low blood pressure when standing and urine retention. Patients are naturally put off by most of these, but if anxiety or agitation is a major accompaniment to the depression, the extra sedation may be beneficial.

SELECTIVE SEROTONIN REUPTAKE INHIBITORS

This other group is also defined by their pharmacological properties, but it is not necessary to know the details of these to understand their clinical use. The selective reuptake inhibitors, now known almost universally as SSRIs, are the most commonly used drugs for depression and now also anxiety, with fluoxetine, sertraline, citalopram, its close relative escitalopram, fluvoxamine and paroxetine being the most widely used. These do not have the anticholinergic side effects of the tricyclic antidepressants but can create nausea, dizziness, diarrhoea, insomnia and sexual dysfunction. Most patients tend to prefer these drugs to the tricyclic antidepressants, partly because they have had much more promotion from the drug industry, but for those who need sedation and improved sleep, the tricyclic group may be superior.

SEROTONIN AND NORADRENALINE REUPTAKE INHIBITORS

These drugs, venlafaxine and duloxetine, have similar adverse effects to the SSRIs. They tend to be used when the SSRIs have been found to lack efficacy. There are other antidepressant drugs, notably mianserin, vortioxetine and mirtazapine, that are somewhat different from the other groups, and this justifies their prescription. There are often used as second-line treatments but some practitioners prefer to use them in place of the other drugs. Agomelatine is a synthetic drug derived from melatonin, a natural substance involved in sleep, that has antidepressant properties. Reboxetine is similar to duloxetine but not prescribed so often.

ANTI-ANXIETY DRUGS

In discussing the separate group of anti-anxiety drugs, it is important to understand that anxiety and depression, although different in nature, are very commonly comorbid; it is useful to remember the couplet 'like wind and rain in stormy weather, these symptoms often come together'. So a primary anti-anxiety drug may be ideal for sedating a depressed patient, and a primary antidepressant drug equally suitable for treating panic and social anxiety. Because of this, it is much better to summarise the use of these drugs by diagnosis, even though there is so much overlap that a combined term, general neurotic syndrome, includes both symptoms equally (Andrews et al., 1990; Tyrer, 2022).

PANIC DISORDER AND AGORAPHOBIA

Panics are sudden, acute episodes of great anxiety occurring for no apparent reason. The person fears that disaster and collapse are imminent, the heart palpitates, breathing becomes difficult and death seems just around the corner. Because these attacks often occur out of doors and in strange places, the patient comes to associate them with being away from home and so avoids going out. This is then called agoraphobia (a word which literally means 'fear of the marketplace' but easily transfers to all situations outside the home).

Although in the past, benzodiazepines were recommended for the treatment of panic, opinions have shifted, and now the preferred drug treatment is one of the SSRIs (see Chapter 13). Panic disorder normally responds very well to psychological treatments to a much greater extent than generalized anxiety disorder.

SOCIAL ANXIETY DISORDER (SOCIAL PHOBIA)

Social anxiety disorder, better shortened as social phobia, shows itself as intense shyness manifest mainly by the belief that others are viewing them negatively in social situations. Because of the anxiety, the feared situations are usually avoided. In this condition as well, both antidepressants such as SSRIs and psychological therapies are effective with no clear superiority shown for either. For acute performance anxiety (e.g. playing a musical instrument solo, public speaking) the needs are different. A drug that reduces the bodily symptoms of anxiety, particularly trembling, such as propranolol or a single dose of a benzodiazepine, may be the only drug needed (Tyrer, 1988).

GENERALIZED ANXIETY DISORDER

This diagnosis is not a very good one as it describes what is left of anxiety when all the other parts have been taken over. It used to be described as 'free-floating anxiety', anxiety that was not attached to any situation or specific stimulus but was there all the time. Benzodiazepine drugs were first recommended for treatment, but as the condition tends to be long-lasting (also see Chapter 7), SSRIs and other antidepressants are now recommended as first-line drug treatments (Craske et al., 2017). However, this is one condition where most patients would fare much better if they were able to access psychological treatments, including mindfulness, relaxation therapy and CBT.

Benzodiazepines may still be used to treat generalized anxiety but ideally only when required in order to avoid dependence. Recently derivatives of gamma-amino butyric acid (GABA) have been introduced, gabapentin and pregabalin. These are effective in treating anxiety, particularly pregabalin, but there is some concern that this particular drug may be addictive. It is certainly well liked by many who have formerly abused drugs, but it would seem wise to use this drug with caution and monitor consumption (Bonnet & Scherbaum, 2017).

OBSESSIONAL DISORDERS

Obsessional disorders, or obsessive-compulsive disorders, with OCD as their common abbreviation, are very well known. The need to think or do something repetitively and uselessly is a bane and a waste of time, a task the sufferer is forced by internal drives to perform. Switching off the need for these rituals is often far from easy. Again, both psychological and drug treatments are of equal effectiveness. The SSRI drugs are specifically recommended, but they may be needed long term.

Tourette's syndrome and tic disorders (abnormal repetitive movements or sounds) are very disturbing disorders found in autism and some behavioural disorders. Tourette's syndrome is the most severe of these and involves both motor (i.e. muscle) twitching and vocal tics (shouts, often of an offensive nature, that the person tries to suppress). Many drugs are recommended for treatment, and this itself suggests that none are ideal. The antipsychotic drugs, haloperidol, and pimozide, are most often used in treatment.

As has also been shown, quite unequivocally, that antidepressants are effective in treating anxiety (Baldwin et al., 2014), the word antidepressant may be outmoded. Although antidepressant effects are largely independent of GABA stimulation, every practitioner needs to be reminded that anxiety and depression are allies in the same concert, not discrete orchestras. What is often treated in practice is mixed anxiety and depression, better termed cothymia (Tyrer, 2001) than mixed anxiety and depressive disorder, which unfortunately can be abbreviated to MADD and is preferably avoided.

Although antipsychotic drugs derived their name, and its synonym, neuroleptic, from their efficacy in schizophrenia, they have definite benefits in the treatment of mood disorders, especially bipolar disorder. Their main use is in the maintenance treatment of bipolar disorder, for which quetiapine, olanzapine and aripiprazole are used; the best results were found with quetiapine, which prevented both manic and depressive episodes (Lindström et al., 2017).

BIPOLAR DISORDER

Bipolar disorder, formerly called manic-depressive psychosis, is a condition affecting about 1% of the population. The condition is called bipolar because it has mania at one pole and depression at the other. Both poles are present in the lifetime of the disorder, but because manic episodes tend to occur first in most cases, once anyone has been demonstrated to have a manic episode, the diagnosis of bipolar disorder is made. You can see that the diagnosis of mania is quite an important issue, and it is worth describing in full.

A manic episode is associated with increased energy, reduced need for sleep, increased sexual drive, a tendency for rapid speech with many changes of direction − commonly called flight of ideas − exaggerated self-worth with grandiose statements about status and greatly elevated mood with euphoria. A manic episode often arises suddenly over the course of one or two days. It often leads to such disruption that admission to hospital is needed. There are often delusions of grandeur and hallucinations in mania, but these are different from those in schizophrenia as they are clearly linked to the increase in mood (i.e. they are mood congruent). Sometimes there are elements of depression mixed with the manic symptoms; this is called a mixed episode of bipolar disorder. The condition called hypomania is essentially the same as mania but at a lower level of intensity.

It is important to emphasise that what is often called 'going manic' in ordinary speech is not clinical mania. Matters have become a little more complicated as in the new ICD-11 classification there is a split between two conditions called bipolar I and bipolar II. Whereas bipolar type I disorder is an episodic mood disorder defined by the occurrence of one or more manic or mixed episodes of depression and mania, bipolar type II disorder is an episodic mood disorder defined by the occurrence of one or more hypomanic episodes and at least one depressive episode. This can be regarded as a useful diagnosis on the bipolar spectrum, but there is a danger that it may lead to confusion with other short-term disorders in which mood swings are prominent. One of these is borderline personality disorder, and as unlike with bipolar disorder, drugs are not particularly of value in treatment, there is a danger that a wrong diagnosis may be followed by the wrong treatment (see Chapter 6).

DRUGS PRIMARILY USED FOR BIPOLAR DISORDER

The most specific drug for bipolar disorder is lithium. This is a single element, quite unlike the complex compounds synthesised in laboratories before extensive testing, and for many years, there was doubt about its value. But there is now unequivocal evidence from trials that it is effective in both preventing manic and hypomanic episodes and also the depressive swings in bipolar disorder (Geddes et al., 2004). But lithium now has to compete with many other drugs, mood stabilisers and antipsychotic drugs in bipolar conditions, and quite often, several drugs may have to be tried before one, or often two, are chosen for treatment.

Lithium is a potentially toxic drug. It has a low therapeutic ratio of 2. The therapeutic ratio is the ratio of the toxic dose and the therapeutic one, and a ratio of 2 indicates that the toxic dose is twice that of the therapeutic one. This is a much lower ratio than most psychotropic drugs and explains why it is necessary to monitor levels of lithium in the blood regularly to keep the blood level between 0.5 and 1.2 (mEql/litre). Lithium is mainly eliminated by the kidneys, and in general those with impaired renal function should not take the drug. It also can impair the uptake of iodine from the gut leading to thyroid deficiency, and this may have to be corrected by taking thyroid hormones.

Many other drugs are taken for bipolar disorder at different stages of the illness. In mania and hypomania, admission to hospital is often necessary as the combination of excessive self-esteem, reckless behaviour, increased energy and overconfidence can put the person in danger or lead to rash decisions that take years to undo. At these times, the patient is psychotic and will need antipsychotic drugs, almost all of which are similarly effective in controlling symptoms.

Lithium is best regarded as a prophylactic drug, one that prevents further episodes of hypomania, mania or depression rather than treating it. In recent years, it has also been shown that some antipsychotic drugs, of which quetiapine is the most used, can also be effective as maintenance drugs in the depressive phase of the bipolar cycle and may be better than specific antidepressant treatment at these times.

POST-TRAUMATIC STRESS DISORDER

Post-traumatic stress disorder is a serious consequence of being exposed to one or more highly traumatic events (e.g. serious accidents, fire, assault). It can also follow repeated exposure to such events in wartime. Drugs are only used at present as supportive agents as the most focused therapies are cognitive behavioural trauma-focused therapy and eye movement for desensitisation reprocessing. But the antidepressants fluoxetine, sertraline, paroxetine and venlafaxine have also been shown to be of value (Mooney et al., 2004; Bisson et al., 2020). The new ICD-11 classification of mental disorders introduces a new condition, complex post-traumatic disorder that applies when the traumatic events occurred many years previously, often in childhood. It is difficult to know if drug treatment may be effective for this condition also.

SLEEP-INDUCING DRUGS (HYPNOTICS)

The purpose of a hypnotic drug is to help sleep. This is one area where there is little confusion between therapist and patient: the word explains the use. Many mental disorders create sleep problems, sometimes too much but more often too little, and drugs given for sleep problems are almost all sedative drugs that promote sleep. These can be divided into several groups for patients to make their choices.

The first group include both prescribed and over-the-counter preparations. These include antihistamines that are primarily used to treat allergies, but many of them have sedative properties, and people who want sedation often buy them without the need for a prescription. These include chlorpheniramine, cinnarizine, diphenhydramine (Nytol), hydroxyzine and promethazine. A full list is in Chapter 13 of this book. They are not classed as addictive, but some people take them long term and have difficulty in stopping them, although not nearly to the same extent as the benzodiazepines.

Sedation is part of the relief of anxiety and promotion of sleep and is found with many drugs which have general sedation as an additional effect, sometimes seen as beneficial but as an unwelcome side effect by others. The drugs promoted particularly for anxiety all act in the same way, mainly by stimulating GABA, a chemical messenger in the brain that when activated has a calming effect. Anxiety is reduced by any drug that stimulates GABA, and, at least when the dosage is right, this reduction of anxiety can be accomplished without sedation. But once this dose is exceeded, there is a general sedative effect, and at higher doses, this leads to loss of consciousness. The best-known GABA-stimulating drugs are the barbiturates, now very seldom used because of their addiction potential; benzodiazepines and what are commonly called the Z-drugs: zopiclone, zolpidem and zaleplon, are primarily used for the treatment of insomnia.

The benzodiazepines are not very different from the Z-drugs. The ones that are marketed primarily as hypnotics are temazepam, flurazepam and nitrazepam. Other drugs that happen to have marked sedation as a side effect are also chosen to aid sleep. These include the tricyclic antidepressants, particularly amitriptyline and trimipramine, and many of the antipsychotic drugs, particularly olanzapine, chlorpromazine and promazine.

The benzodiazepines and Z-drugs all act as GABA-stimulating drugs and in somewhat lower dosage have anxiety-reducing effects. The pharmaceutical companies like to identify a 'hole in the market' when they are introducing new compounds, and a great deal of research goes into finding where these holes are. So if there appears to be an increasing market for a new hypnotic drug, it is very simple to move a drug from the position of relieving anxiety to one of inducing sleep; you just market it at a higher dose. Other factors also come into play, including the presence of other mental illness, so for example, a depressed patient with marked insomnia may be prescribed a tricyclic antidepressant to cover both sleep and antidepressant requirements. The sedative effects of antidepressants and antipsychotic drugs are more complex and not so specific as the benzodiazepines and Z-drugs and tend to have more side effects.

The decision to take a hypnotic drug for the first time should not be taken lightly. A normal good night's sleep is best described by Shakespeare in *Macbeth*: it not only knits up the ravelled sleeve of care, acts as a balm for the troubled mind and is a key nourisher of life's feast but also allows the sleeper to awake refreshed, alert and well set to face the challenges of the day. A drug-induced sleep, even with the best of chemicals, never approaches this level of performance. There is a vast literature on the gloomy subject called 'the residual effects of hypnotics', but the simple fact is that no effective hypnotic is completely free from the effects of brain fog, headache and head swimming, daze and continued drowsiness on waking.

As such, it is always reasonable to question whether a hypnotic drug is needed at all. The manufacturers of the night-time drink Ovaltine® increased their sales markedly when a kind researcher reported that the drink contained a significant quantity of the element magnesium, which is mildly sedative. Avoiding coffee and other high-caffeine-containing drinks in the evening and before going to bed also helps to promote natural sleep.

But there are many situations when it is unwise to be puritanical and better to take a safe hypnotic drug than suffer persistent insomnia. The continuing presence of pain and other symptoms despite taking analgesics makes many dread the thought of going to bed when its anticipation should be one of the most welcoming parts of the day. A hypnotic drug can at least partially offset this discomfort. Similarly, insomnia after a major and unexpected event can be very troubling, and here, there is the expectation that the drug may only be needed for a few days.

One drug, melatonin, reinforces the body's reaction to darkness by inducing sleep. It is produced by the pineal gland in the brain and is secreted at dusk. The consequence is that our body clocks are kept in time with the hours of daylight and explains why we sleep longer in the winter months than in the summer. Melatonin in a modified release form can be taken once daily in the evenings for resistant insomnia. It is also used by passengers on long-distance east–west flights to help in adjusting to time zones.

Hypnotic drugs have a chequered history of harm. It has been known for centuries that sedative drugs such as opiates can be fatal in overdosage. When the only drugs available were barbiturates, and more commonly in hospitals, chloral hydrate, the initial views were that they were safer than their predecessors. This was premature, and before long the number of deaths due to barbiturate overdosage (and to cardiac and respiratory deaths with chloral) steadily rose. It was also not fully appreciated that even a therapeutic dose of a barbiturate can be accentuated by alcohol into a fatal overdose. Marilyn Monroe, at a time in her life when all was relatively stable – she had just bought a new house and was modifying it in her own unusual style – died from an apparent overdose, but almost certainly an accidental poisoning from alcohol and barbiturates combined.

When the benzodiazepines were introduced and demonstrated to be much safer than the barbiturates, there was a dramatic shift which when combined with campaigns to stop taking barbiturates led to a massive change in prescriptions for these new apparently wonder drugs. They were safe in overdosage, seemingly effective in inducing sleep with relatively few after-effects, and they made everyone happy, especially the manufacturers of these new compounds.

Then the problem of withdrawal symptoms in therapeutic dosage became known (discussed in more detail later), and recommendations were made for short-term prescription only. But this was not a particular safety issue, and we should still remember that when taken alone, all benzodiazepines are very safe drugs; it is when they are combined with other sedative drugs or alcohol that they become problems. It also should be noted that safety at home is not the same as safety when travelling; benzodiazepine consumption increases the risk of traffic accidents (Skegg et al., 1979). Most hypnotic drugs act quickly and sleepiness is noted within an hour. The Z-drugs are particularly known for their rapid speed of action and some people find that they should take their dose immediately before going to bed, as it is said that if people take them too early in the evening they may fall asleep on the stairs.

ADVERSE EFFECTS

The main adverse effect of all hypnotic drugs can be summarised as accentuated hangovers. The combination of muzziness, difficulty in concentration, drowsiness and brain fog are all due to the drug continuing its action when it is no longer desired. Other adverse effects are less common; they include gastrointestinal disturbance (nausea, vomiting, diarrhoea), dizziness and dry mouth, more marked with the antidepressant and antipsychotic drugs.

ANTIDEPRESSANT DRUGS FOR OTHER BODILY CONDITIONS

There are a very large number of conditions that are treated with antidepressant drugs, but it is far from clear whether this is only because depression may be such a common part of other syndromes. When a drug is found that helps any mental symptom its use can very easily be extended to other conditions inappropriately. This is where some of the criticisms of excessive drug use by Joanna Moncrieff and others have some justification. So if insomnia is part of any chronic disorder such as arthritis and other painful conditions, or conditions such as irritable bowel syndrome, what are often called medically unexplained symptoms or somatic disorders, become persistent, and antidepressant is frequently prescribed. If it is effective, it may only be treating the depressive component of the disorder. Despite this uncertainty, formal recommendations are made for antidepressants to be used in these conditions (Vasant et al., 2021).

DRUGS FOR ALCOHOL PROBLEMS

Alcohol problems constitute a spectrum of illness that is often unrecognised as so much alcohol excess is hidden by those who are addicted. The two areas where drugs are most frequently used are in the detoxification of alcohol dependence and in preventing the excessive use of alcohol.

DETOXIFICATION

A patient with addiction to alcohol is unable to have any significant periods in the day when they are not drinking. Those who only drink to excess at weekends are not addicted. Detoxification becomes necessary when alcohol consumption is completely out of control and both the patient and relatives or friends see withdrawal as a necessary part of any recovery.

The most common drugs used to assist alcohol withdrawal are the benzodiazepines, particularly chlordiazepoxide, better known by most as Librium. Clormethiazole (clomethiazole) is a drug closer to the barbiturates that is similar in effectiveness in enabling alcohol reduction but has a greater risk of dependence. There are many regimes describing the detoxification from alcohol, but they all adopt a dosing strategy with drugs such as diazepam and chlordiazepoxide, using either a rating scale triggered by symptoms so that more of the benzodiazepine is given when symptoms increase (Elholm et al., 2011) or a fixed-dose withdrawal schedule with gradual reduction over 5–14 days (Lingford-Hughes et al., 2012). Carbamazepine, most commonly used as a mood stabiliser in bipolar disorder, also has some efficacy as an additional treatment during alcohol withdrawal (Hammond et al., 2015). GABAs may also be useful in withdrawal but at present cannot be recommended (Hammond et al., 2015).

PREVENTION OF RETURN TO ALCOHOL

Once a dependent patient has stopped taking alcohol, it is often a hard task to prevent a return. Organisations such as Alcoholics Anonymous are very good in this area, and the group pressure that can applied, often not perceived as pressure but highly effective, can probably carry out this form of management better than any drug. But there is one drug, acamprosate, that has been shown to be effective in preventing a return to alcohol, and unlike other drugs, it does not have any serious side effects and is not prone to dependence (Sinclair et al., 2016).

Naltrexone and nalmifene are opiate antagonists (i.e. they block the pleasurable sensations of opiates) and are also of some value in reducing alcohol consumption. Naltrexone is the stronger of the two in blocking the effects of alcohol. Nalmefene seems to work more by reducing the unpleasant consequences of alcohol withdrawal.

Disulfiram was the original drug used to prevent return to alcohol. It is a drug that prevents the full breakdown of alcohol in the body so that one of its metabolites, acetaldehyde, accumulates in the body, creating unpleasant flushing, headache, nausea and vomiting with a fall in blood pressure. This can be fatal if much alcohol is consumed. Disulfiram is less often used today.

Acamprosate is a more favoured drug to prevent return to drinking. It is an unusual drug in having very few interactions with other drugs and may also be safe in overdosage. It is also not likely to be abused (Sinclair et al., 2016), so it has the potential to be used more often. Baclofen, a drug used for the treatment of spasticity, may also have a place in preventing a return to drinking (Agabio et al., 2023) and is used in many countries more often than in the United Kingdom.

PSYCHOSTIMULANTS

Only two psychostimulant drugs are currently recommended in mental health practice, methylphenidate and lisdexamfetamine, both for the treatment of attention deficit hyperactivity disorder (ADHD). Three drugs that are not stimulants, atomoxetine, bupriopion and guanfacine, are also prescribed if patients cannot tolerate psychostimulants. Methylphenidate and lisdexamfetine (the latter derived from the original psychostimulant, amphetamine) are both controlled drugs, prescriptions of which are carefully monitored and which require oversight. At first sight, it seems odd that drugs that increased nervous activity in the brain are valuable in the treatment of a condition characterised by impulsive behaviour, a poor attention span and great distractibility should be helped by stimulants. When the positive effects on this behaviour in children were reported by Charles Bradley in 1937, few people could believe these drugs were effective, and it took many years before others repeated his study and confirmed the findings.

Nonetheless, despite the now unequivocal evidence that stimulants are effective in treating ADHD, supported by over 100 randomized trials (Cortese et al., 2018), there continue to be arguments about the value of drugs for this condition. Psychological treatment of childhood mental health problems seems to be a natural choice, but there is also considerable argument about the utility of the diagnosis of ADHD (Moncrieff & Timimi, 2010).

All the drugs I have listed are superior to placebo tablets and can be justified for treatment, but caution is merited in prescribing stimulant drugs; especially in young people, doing so needs a full explanation and agreement before starting therapy. But today, we are not just thinking about psychostimulant for ADHD but apparently are on the brink of a massive change in psychiatric practice, the psychedelic revolution (Nutt, 2023), with renewed interest in the first psychedelic, psilocybin. The drugs in this group are not yet available on prescription and are unlikely to appear for some time.

Psychostimulants, when effective, which is true of most cases, reduce all the symptoms and abnormal behaviour of ADHD; attention increases, distractibility and impulsiveness decrease and concentration is maintained to a much greater extent than before. All these improvements tend to occur together and often the change is dramatic. The phenomenon of tolerance – less effect after repeated dosage – is rarely found with psychostimulants. Because in schoolchildren the problems of distractibility and difficult behaviour are often shown primarily at school, it is common for drug holidays at weekends to be allowed, although there is uncertain evidence of its value in maintaining treatment regularly on other days. Psychedelic drugs have received much attention recently, but as none are clinically available, they are not included in this book, but might appear in a later edition.

Patient questions answered

What are these drugs? They are all drugs that increase activation in the brain.

Is it safe? When prescribed and taken properly, they are very safe. Their main problems are that they can easily be abused.

Do they have side effects? Yes, the most common ones are an increase in blood pressure, nausea, increased nervousness and sleep problems if taken late in the day (not with guanfacine and atomoxetine).

Exactly when do I expect benefit and how long should I take them for? They start acting immediately, and change is usually notice within a day. There is no fixed period of treatment, and medication can be extended from childhood into adult life.

DRUGS FOR COMPULSIVE SEXUAL BEHAVIOUR

Compulsive sexual behaviour is now a formal diagnosis, and its diagnostic limits need to be tested. It is most common in men. Oestradiol and progesterone-like agents are sometimes of value in this condition. The antipsychotic drug benperidol has also been promoted for this and for the management of paedophilia, but its claims for effectiveness are slim (Landgren et al., 2022).

DRUGS FOR ERECTILE DYSFUNCTION

Erectile dysfunction is not often written about in prescribing practice. Some claim it is not a disorder as it does not interfere with ordinary life, but it does. It is not a psychological addendum to normal living but a diagnosis pointing to the presence of a bodily problem, and, as such, is perfectly appropriate for drug therapy. Because of a combination of embarrassment, stigma and reticence, it has only just been recognised to have a greater incidence than most other diseases. Note the word 'disease'. Erectile impotence and osteoarthritis are almost equally common, and both are diseases in that they prevent normal function, in other words, increase morbidity. They are also linked strongly to age.

A recent review of the incidence of erectile dysfunction in all studies available at that time (2013) showed figures of 6% in men aged 40–49, 16% aged 50–59, 32% aged 60–69 and 44% aged 70–79 (Eardley, 2013). The difference in successful therapies between osteoarthritis and erectile dysfunction is considerable. Most osteoarthritis requires surgery that can often prove complicated; erectile dysfunction just requires a single tablet, soon to be replaced by topical agents. With nearly half of elderly men having erectile dysfunction, with much higher proportions in those with diabetes, it is not surprising that the first drug to treat the condition, sildenafil, was the fastest-selling drug in history when it was launched in 1998, and it has generated annual sales of £1.4 billion ever since.

The person who deserves most credit for making erectile dysfunction a medical disorder is Giles Brindley, a highly intelligent enterprising researcher who revels in lateral thinking. He edited the first book I wrote (Tyrer, 1976), and his many scribblings in the margins of my text helped to make the book a much better final product. He was the first to demonstrate that erectile dysfunction could be treated by drugs (Brindley, 1983) by injecting a drug, phenoxybenzamine, which blocks the effect of adrenoceptors (adrenaline receptors) on the muscles that keep the penis small, so that then it becomes erect and tumescent. As an active experimenter, he had tested this drug, and indeed many others, on himself before treating any patients.

What was unusual was the way in which he demonstrated this discovery to the world. At an evening public lecture in Las Vegas in 1983, he appeared in a blue track suit, not really appropriate for a formal occasion. This was tolerated by his American hosts as he was clearly an English eccentric and so could be excused. But he had a reason for his attire. He had injected his penis with another drug, papaverine, before the lecture, which can maintain an erection for several hours. While giving the lecture he suddenly dropped his track suit bottoms to expose his erect penis and walked off the stage to pass through the audience below, asking them to confirm by touch that his penis was firmly erect and there was no simulation in place. A few of the female members of the audience gave strangulated screams, others stared fascinated, but Giles continued until he was satisfied that enough touching had taken place and the feelers could not find a penile prosthesis anywhere.

Some may think this was an unnecessarily flamboyant way of demonstrating a scientific discovery, but I think this stand-up lecture by Giles had a much bigger impact than any number of scientific articles in learned journals and showed to the world that erectile impotence was as much a medical subject as the psychoanalyst's couch. It was the stimulus that led to the development of Viagra. The two drugs currently available on prescription, sildenafil (the original Viagra) and tadalafil (Cialis), are taken by mouth just before sexual intercourse. (There is no need for injections now.) Both have relatively few adverse effects and do not need to be given in repeat dosage.

OFF-LABEL PRESCRIBING

One of the important reasons for linking diagnosis to prescribed drugs is that each drug is licensed for one or more named diagnoses, either named specifically or as a general group. This does not mean that the prescriber cannot prescribe the drug for other conditions, but the practice has to be identified clearly and justification given. When drugs are given for another unapproved condition, the prescription is defined as 'off-label'. When a drug is prescribed for an approved condition but is given in a higher dose than approved, in a different formulation (e.g. liquid) or in an age group excluded from ordinary prescription, these are also off-label prescriptions. In a good prescriber partnership, off-label prescribing will be disclosed to the patient and the special reasons for its prescription given. If patients object and refuse the prescription in an off-label form, they have absolute right to do so.

For those who are interested in a fuller account of the effectiveness of drugs and other treatments in psychiatric disorders linked to diagnosis, a full account can be found elsewhere (Tyrer & Silk, 2008; Taylor et al., 2021). There is also a summary version (Tyrer & Silk, 2011). For those who would like fuller information about the mechanisms of psychotropic drug action, please look at *Seminars in Clinical Psychopharmacology*, edited by Peter Haddad and David Nutt (2020). In examining the value of different drugs, it is important to look at independent reviews as those that are in any way sponsored by the drug industry tend to show at least some evidence of bias.

CENTRAL MESSAGES OF CHAPTER 5

1. When a prescription for a psychotropic drug is being given, both prescriber and patient should be clear for what condition it is being prescribed for, with at least a vague indication of the diagnosis.

2. For many disorders, specific psychological treatments are as effective as drugs; patients should always have the option of choice.

6

PERSONALITY AND DRUG TREATMENT

This might seem to be an unusual chapter. Other books on drug treatment have very little to say about personality, but we should take notice of it. All of us have distinct personalities, and these should influence how we take drugs and for how long. This statement may appear odd at first. Surely a drug is being given to counteract symptoms of stress and distress, or to treat severe mental illness: what has that got to do with personality? There are many answers to this question, but first we need to clarify what personality is and how it influences our lives.

PERSONALITY IS A MOTIVATING FORCE

What we do in life, what makes us happy or discontented; what makes us ambitious or indifferent and what determines our work, relationships and satisfaction ultimately depends on personality. The essential you that separates you from others is your personality. When Oscar Wilde wrote wittily, 'be yourself, everyone else is taken', he was putting forward a universal truth. You are a unique individual, and at the centre of this special person is your personality.

Taking a drug is an important event for your personality. Are you taking it as a crutch or prop to keep you on a level keel, a booster to your energy and performance, or a desperate attempt to keep afloat in a sea of troubles? Behind the answers to these questions is your personality.

Your personality is unique, but this does not mean it cannot be broken down or analysed. In the latest classification of personality problems (ICD-11), all people are on a single dimension of personality,

DOI: 10.1201/9781032619019-7

and the five main areas (called domains) have unusual names but describe common characteristics. These are 'negative affective' (translated roughly as nervous gloom-mongers), 'dissocial' (antisocial and egotistical), 'anankastic' (fussy and methodical), 'disinhibited' (reckless and impulsive) and detached (isolated and avoiders of company) (Tyrer et al., 2019). We all have at least a smidgeon of one or more of these characteristics, which affects our attitudes and our reactions to drugs.

For example, I am somewhat anankastic (obsessional) in that I do not like the idea of any drug having any control over my feelings, so I try to avoid psychotropic drugs wherever possible. If I were compelled to take them for any reason, I would like them to be stopped as soon as possible. The last thing I would expect is to be dependent on them.

PERSONALITY IS THE MAIN REASON BEHIND CHOICE IN LIFE

When you consider the pathways taken in life, they may at first seem to be a combination of fate and random occurring in sequence. Yes, we can all turn to single experiences and say they changed the course of your life, but when you look at them more closely, there is a trend linked very closely to personality. We follow where our personality leads us, even if we do not recognise it. Fate and circumstance play a part, but they do not control our destinies. The people we choose to spend our lives with, the occupations we take up, the places where we live, the friends with whom we spend comfortable times, the sports and leisure activities we take up are all a combination of abilities and preferences steered by our personalities.

PERSONALITY ATTITUDES TO DRUG TREATMENT

The same factors that guide us through life also apply to our attitudes and responses to drugs. If we take a simple example, the attitude toward a painkiller such as paracetamol, we can see a pattern. Those like me who have a strong need to control our lives and will only take paracetamol or another painkiller when the pain is very intense. At other times, we put up with it – I argue that by knowing the pain is still present I can understand its course and progress better – whereas if I took painkillers regularly, I would not know what is really going on inside.

If I am a demanding and impulsive soul, I look for instant relief whenever anything unpleasant happens and so will take painkillers readily, often exceeding the prescribed dose if I do not get rapid benefit. If I am a worrier who sees disaster around every corner, I am very sensitive to the effects of painkillers; I cannot tolerate the pain and so take the tablets exactly as recommended on the pack but monitor my pain carefully and make sure I have enough tablets available if I have to take them long term. I am acutely aware of variation in the pain and worry even more if it does not seem to be getting better. Detached personalities are often described as stoical; they do not bother too much with minor disabilities. They will take painkillers, but almost as an afterthought, and certainly will not be waiting by the clock to take their next dose. These may appear to be stereotypes but there is truth in all of them.

When it comes to taking psychotropic drugs, the same principles apply. Your personality determines to what extent you will follow the advice on your prescription. Some will take their medication assiduously; at the other extreme, some will follow Macbeth's admonition in Shakespeare's play – 'throw physic to the dogs. I'll none of it' – and hardly take any at all, and others will miss out doses at different times when there seems to be more important things to do. You can anticipate this as a prescriber if you know something about the patient you are treating. You may not want to bring the word 'personality' into your decision, but it is there hovering in the background.

BORDERLINE PERSONALITY DISORDER

Although those with disorders of personality, particularly borderline personality disorder, are often treated with drugs, there is no good evidence they are effective (Stoffers-Winterling et al., 2022). Despite this, borderline, or emotionally unstable personality disorder as it is diagnosed in the United Kingdom at present, is often treated with not just one but two or three psychotropic drugs. In a recent study of UK practice, 92% of all patients with emotionally unstable personality disorder were taking one or more psychotropic drugs (Paton et al., 2015).

Why this large proportion while those with other personality disorders rarely receive treatment? The reason is that borderline personality disorder presents primarily with distressing symptoms – anger, anxiety, suicidal feelings and despair – immediate relief is desired. Other personality disorders are based on exaggeration of common traits that are present in all of us. I, and many others, do not think borderline (emotionally unstable) is a personality disorder at all, as it is so different from other disorders and also overlaps with many other conditions (which explains its name), and consequently is far too widely diagnosed (Mulder & Tyrer, 2023).

In the new classification of personality disorder, the borderline option is not a diagnosis; it is called a 'pattern specifier', a term needing a wordsmith to analyse. The problem is that anyone who gets involved in an argument, loses their temper and storms off but feels bad afterwards can satisfy the borderline epithet. If this label is attached, it becomes a toxic one, leading to the assumption that patients with the condition are unreliable, difficult, argumentative and to be avoided. This all contributes to making the diagnosis grossly stigmatising.

But this does not mean that the central component of the diagnosis, emotional dysregulation, does not exist. It is a very unpleasant symptom, but unlike true personality disorders, is not a persistent trait that permanently affects behaviour. It has a good outcome in the long run, but in the short term it is often treated with drugs. So why is it treated so often with drugs, increasingly so in adolescents who often take up to three different drugs a day, mainly antidepressants and tranquillizers?

It does not take much to guess what happens in a typical prescriber/patient interaction. Emotional turmoil is devastatingly unpleasant, instant relief is desired, only a drug will suffice: the patient must leave the clinic with a prescription. But if this only takes the edge off the symptoms (e.g., through sedation), the patient comes back and asks for more. 'The other tablets seem to have worn off, doctor, but I don't want to stop them yet. Can I have something else to back them up?' And so the merry-go-round of prescription goes on.

All drugs prescribed for borderline or emotionally unstable personality disorder are off-label, at every age, in whatever dosage and for however long.

PERSONALITY AND PROBLEMS OF WITHDRAWAL

You might think that personality has very little to do with the complex issue of withdrawal from psychotropic drugs. If all withdrawal problems were directly related to addiction and dependent on the pharmacological properties of the drug, personality would have very little place in influencing withdrawal. But as you can see from other chapters in this book, withdrawal problems are not straightforward and depend on many factors including psychological ones. If you are a pessimist and expect problems in every aspect of life, then you are much more likely to be worried about withdrawing from psychotropic drugs. You will be more likely to take notice of problems of withdrawal from media outlets, friends and relatives, and so you will be sensitive to withdrawal effects. These personality features are prominent in the negative affective domain of personality. Worriers have more problems reducing drugs than non-worriers.

If on the other hand you are like me and do not like taking drugs unless it is absolutely necessary, the process of withdrawal is embraced with enthusiasm. Any symptoms that might be thought of as distressing are tolerated readily as the patient cannot wait to be free of these mind-altering drugs that complicate all sorts of decision-making. In between we have the detached personalities who are largely indifferent to withdrawal problems and also cope with them well if they arise. The other group who might have difficulty in withdrawal are those with impulsive personalities who tend to exaggerate both positive and negative problems in life. If these people experience withdrawal symptoms, the symptoms are immediately seen as alarming and some sort of action has to be taken.

These statements, although they face validity (i.e., they seem to make sense), need backing up with evidence. Evidence exists, and I will describe one part of it in full. When we carried out a study of gradual benzodiazepine withdrawal (Tyrer et al., 1983), described more fully in the next chapter, we also recorded personality characteristics before any withdrawal took place, using the Personality Assessment Schedule (Tyrer & Alexander, 1979; Tyrer et al., 1979; Tyrer, 2022). This interview asks about the presence and intensity of 24 personality attributes. The scores range from 0 to 8, with 0 indicating complete absence of the characteristic and 8 indicating such intensity of the attribute that it dominates behaviour (and can only be given for one of the 24 items).

After the trial had been completed, we compared the personality profiles of those who had had withdrawal symptoms with those who did not have withdrawal problems. The separation of those with withdrawal symptoms was an increase in symptoms of 50% or the presence of two new symptoms during withdrawal. Thirty-six patients completed the trial, and of these, 16 had withdrawal symptoms and 20 did not.

In analysing the results, I need to emphasise that this was a small study, and too much should not be concluded definitively from the findings. But when you look at the differences in personality between those who had withdrawal problems and those who did not, the findings back up what I have written earlier in this chapter. The worried, anxious pessimists who expect trouble around every corner are well represented in the withdrawal group. Those with high scores on emotional lability, anxiousness and resourcelessness were much more likely to have withdrawal symptoms. Similarly, those who scored high on impulsiveness and irresponsibility also had higher rates of withdrawal symptoms. There was also some indication that those who worried about their health (hypochondriacs, whom we would now say have health anxiety) also had higher withdrawal problems.

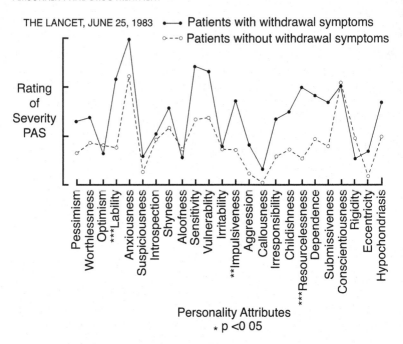

Figure 6.1   Personality differences between patients with and without withdrawal symptoms in trial of gradual withdrawal of diazepam. PAS = Personality Assessment Schedule. (From Tyrer et al. 1983.)

Although little notice was taken of this finding when it was published, it has had a considerable impact in the longer term. The same findings were shown in two further studies (Schweizer et al., 1998; Tönne et al., 1998), and this led to the British National Formulary noting this in its advice about benzodiazepines: 'personality disorder (within the fearful group – dependent, avoidant, obsessive-compulsive) may increase risk of dependence'. In the new ICD-11 classification of personality disorder (Tyrer et al., 2021), this will need to change to 'mild or moderate personality disorder with prominent domain scores in negative affectivity and additional dependence may increase the risk of dependence'.

When the first reports of benzodiazepine dependence began to appear in the literature, there was an excited rustling in the quiet halls of the legal profession as there was a strong possibility that class action could be taken against drug companies on the grounds that they knew of the potential for dependence but intentionally withheld this information from doctors. This was indeed initiated and was the biggest class action in UK history: it involved 14,000 patients and 1,800 law firms. No decision was ever reached, and legal aid was withdrawn once the deadlock became clear.

I do not know all the reasons the class action failed, but the data sheets of the drug companies that accompany all new drugs stated that benzodiazepines should not be given to those with personality disorder. This may have been on the basis of evidence that the companies had from their own studies or may have been a general protective clause. Whatever the reason, the evidence from our own studies that personality factors were relevant in the withdrawal syndrome must have helped their defence.

But in 1983, we had no extra knowledge to guide us. The only conclusion that we could possibly make from these findings was that personality factors were a major predictor of withdrawal problems. This was a surprising conclusion, as our reason for adding the personality assessment to the study was one of curiosity: the subject had not been previously addressed, and at the time we never expected any important differences in personality to be shown.

This finding has had a major influence on my own prescribing ever since 1983. Even though I cannot make a full assessment of personality status in every patient I see, I try to get a good idea of the facets of obsessionality, impulsiveness, dependence, sensitivity and anxiousness in all of them and give advice accordingly. The full advice I give comes in a comprehensive explanation in the last chapter of this book, but I give some examples below of how I have used personality status in making clinical decisions.

EXAMPLE 1

Mr Brown was an accountant with a well-known international firm. He had always been highly competent at his job but found as he came into his fifties that he was getting increasingly anxious about making decisions in case he made a major error. He spent many hours cross-checking his work and did not find anything more than minor mistakes, but this was not enough reassurance and did not stop him checking. He had seen a number of doctors and had taken benzodiazepines, which he rejected almost immediately as he felt sleepy and found they impaired his performance; then he was treated with two different antidepressants, the first a tricyclic that made him sleep too much left him constipated and the second an SSRI that he found he could tolerate but that had no real impact on his anxiety.

When I saw him, he was asking for further medication as he had no wish to have psychological treatment for his anxiety. His antagonism to psychological treatment was not well founded, but he was adamant that this should not be pursued. After a full assessment, I prescribed him the MAOI phenelzine at a dose of 15 mg twice daily with the intention of raising the dose later. Why did I choose this drug? It was partly because I had a lot of experience with the drug and often found that it was highly effective if treatment continued for long enough (Tyrer et al., 1980). The other reason was that I had assessed his basic personality status without too much difficulty and realized that he would be absolutely careful about observing all the requirements of people taking this class of drugs.

The last point is particularly important. The MAOIs were the first antidepressants to be marketed, but their popularity suffered a major blow when it was found that the substance tyramine, found in ripe cheeses such as blue cheese or Stilton, when taken with these drugs led to a sudden and sometimes catastrophic rise in blood pressure (Blackwell & Mabbitt, 1965). This was because tyramine raises the blood pressure, but under normal circumstances it is broken down in the body immediately and has no effect. Not all people get this 'cheese reaction' as it is often caused, as there are other ways in which tyramine is broken down, but it has major implications. Other foods such as cured meats, very ripe fruit such as bananas and oranges, young broad beans (especially pods) and fermented wines (sherry, vermouth) all have high tyramine content and should be avoided.

What is more, other antidepressants and even some antihistamines (e.g. chlorpheniramine) interact in a similar way and lead to a rise in blood pressure. Pharmacists are fully aware of all these drug and dietary dangers, and a warning leaflet is given to all patients once they are prescribed. When choosing who might be treated with an MAOI, the prescriber needs to have a reliable, some might say obsessional, patient who would follow all the food and drug restrictions to the letter.

My accountant was just this kind of person. He took a sort of perverse pleasure in giving me the details of his regular diet, and it was clear that he was not a fan of the banned foods. He responded very well to his prescription (after three and a half weeks as there is often some delay), his anxiety was greatly reduced and his energy and confidence enhanced. He continued on the same dose of phenelzine until he retired a few years later. His personality structure was a major reason leading to my prescription. MAOIs are not used very often today, but when patients' anxiety and depressive symptoms have failed to respond to all the well-known drugs, prescribing a drug such as phenelzine (most commonly), tranylcypromine (the most powerful), or isocarboxazid (the safest), is worthy of consideration in a small selection of people.

EXAMPLE 2

Miss White was a secretary who had just been referred to the GP from the Accident & Emergency (A&E) department of her local hospital. She had recently had an acute episode of pain in the chest, breathlessness and fears of dying while on her way to work. At the A&E department, it was feared she might have had a heart attack, but all tests were normal, and it was concluded that she had had a panic attack. It was felt further assessment and referral might be necessary, so she had been referred to her GP, who felt a psychiatric assessment was needed.

When I saw her, she was relatively calm, but she did describe two further panic episodes since the major one. In my further enquiry into her background, she acknowledged a tendency to be anxious when faced with any new situation and disclosed that both her mother and maternal grandmother had been highly nervous people, with her grandmother rarely going outside her cottage for the last 20 years of her life because of agoraphobia. When asked about treatment preferences, she said she had a slight preference for some form of psychological treatment rather than drugs as 'I don't want to get dependent on them'.

After discussion about other life circumstances – she had just been married and was thinking of having a baby – we came to a conclusion: 'because of your personal constitution and background, I think you would have difficulties stopping any of the standard drugs used for treating panic and it would be wise to avoid them. Instead I am going to refer you to a clinical psychologist who is an expert in CBT for those with panic and she normally completes her treatment in only six sessions. Would you be happy with this suggestion?' This was accepted readily, and she responded well to treatment, as indeed do most people (Clark et al., 1999): panic disorder is the most appropriate common mental disorder to treat with CBT. It also has a better long-term outcome than most other anxiety or depressive disorders (Tyrer et al., 2022).

It is not difficult to see how Miss White's personality status was a major factor in choosing the right therapy for her symptoms of panic. Her genetic and personal history would make it highly likely that she would have difficulty in stopping both benzodiazepines and antidepressants if either had been prescribed. CBT for panic symptoms takes longer to relieve symptoms than drug treatment, but because there was not a desperate need for symptomatic relief, she was quite happy to wait for appointments for treatment. Since 2005, talking treatments, mainly CBT, are available for all anxiety disorders (Nice, 2011), and the main problem at present is the long waiting time before appointments are given.

It was also relevant that Miss White was thinking of getting pregnant. There is a great deal of concern about the damaging effects of drugs on the unborn infant – some drugs such as valproate, carbamazepine and lithium should be avoided in any patient who is pregnant or thinking of pregnancy – and not all others can be given a complete bill of health as it sometimes takes many years before the risks are identified. One only needs to mention thalidomide, first prescribed as a hypnotic, to appreciate this.

For many people, the idea of a personality assessment is forbidding, requiring hours of assessment. This is not true. A very short scale, the Structured Assessment of Personality – Abbreviated Scale (Moran et al., 2003), has only eight questions about sociability, trust in others, impulsiveness and temper, worry, obsessionality and dependence and can be accessed online. It is only a screen for personality disturbance but is a pretty good one. It could be used regularly in GP surgeries. It is the mark of a well-rounded practitioner to assess personality status in a patient. A therapeutic conclusion that combines understanding of symptoms, predispositions and personality strengths and weaknesses is more likely to be a sound one than an assessment of symptoms alone.

MESSAGES FROM CHAPTER 6

1.   If you are a patient, take the trouble to analyse your own personality and how it affects your views on drug treatment.

2.   If you are a prescriber, do not be afraid to address the issue of personality with your patients, including formal assessments, as it could be important in choosing treatments.

7

THE SPECIAL PROBLEM OF BENZODIAZEPINES

The late Richard Asher, a noted physician who first pointed out the dangers of bed rest as a medical prescription and introduced the name Munchausen's syndrome to the range of conditions now called 'factitious psychosis', was very hot on the proper use of language. In one piece of correspondence, he took issue with another doctor who contradicted one of Asher's assertions in a letter. His colleague started it by saying, 'it is well known that X is a cause of Y'. Asher replied by writing, 'I agree it is well known that X is a cause of Y; the mistake he makes is believing that what is well known is therefore true.'

I list below nine statements about benzodiazepines that are also well known and in not being true are actually misleading. Each of these has been made in different places but reinforced by different groups around the world who are campaigning against the use of benzodiazepines. The most active in the United States is called the Benzodiazepine Information Coalition, and the UK one is Benzo.org.uk with a subtitle: The resource site for involuntary benzodiazepine tranquillizer addiction, withdrawal and recovery. A substantial part of the information on the website is the Ashton Manual, reproduced in the website in full and written by the late Heather Ashton, a pharmacologist from Newcastle-on-Tyne.

This campaign has been supported by many MPs (responding to their constituents' concerns) and the then Prime Minister, now Lord Cameron, Foreign Secretary, acknowledged the size of the problem in the House of Commons in 2013: 'First, I pay tribute to the Hon. Gentleman (Jim Dobbin, MP), who has campaigned strongly on this issue over many years. I join him in paying tribute to Professor Ashton, whom I know has considerable expertise in this area. He is right to say that this is a terrible affliction; these people are not drug addicts but they have become hooked on repeat prescriptions of tranquillizers.

DOI: 10.1201/9781032619019-8

The Minister for Public Health is very happy to discuss this issue with him and, as he says, make sure that the relevant guidance can be issued'.

Because a great deal of attention has been given to the Ashton Manual (last version published in 2002), it is appropriated to examine this carefully. In doing this I should say that I knew Heather Ashton well (she died in 2019), partly because she was a good friend of my twin brother, Stephen, who worked in an office next to her in Newcastle. In my criticisms of some of the content of the Ashton Manual, I want to emphasise that I have a very high regard for her work in this area as she was one of the few people who did not just tub-thump about the dangers of benzodiazepines but muscled down and saw a large number of people who were having great difficulty in coming off their drugs and who had no-one else to turn to.

The problem I have when reading the Ashton Manual is that its general tenor is almost all about the dangers of the benzodiazepines, not their benefits. True, as she was a highly esteemed pharmacologist, she knew the subject well and acknowledges the benefits of these drugs – 'few drugs can compete with them in efficacy, rapid onset of action and low acute toxicity (Ashton M, Chapter 1)' – but all her work in the area was focused on withdrawal, not the treatment of mental illness. She was not a psychiatrist and so did not treat patients who presented with anxiety and were helped by benzodiazepines, so none of the advice in the Ashton Manual gives more than a passing nod to their benefits in the longer term. Many of her statements and her recommendations have been taken up by the activists in organisations helping tranquillizer addiction, sometimes a little out of context, and some of them come into the 'well-known but false' categories of Richard Asher.

IT IS WELL KNOWN THAT BENZODIAZEPINES SHOULD ONLY BE GIVEN FOR TWO TO FOUR WEEKS AND THEN WITHDRAWN

This advice, reproduced by most official bodies, is compounded by a second statement from Benzo.org.uk that 'People taking benzodiazepines regularly long term (longer than 2 to 4 weeks) may have symptoms of withdrawal even when they have not reduced the dose'. This addition is understandable as the phenomenon of tolerance (the effect of the drug becoming less after repeated dosage) is very rapid after taking a benzodiazepine, so it is possible to argue that the anti-anxiety effect is less, but it is a step further to imply that any increase in anxiety is de facto a withdrawal symptom.

This fallacy about short-term use is not just stated by campaign groups but by almost every national authority on the subject, including NICE and the British National Formulary (the official consensus of drugs in the United Kingdom). The reason it is wrong is that *regular* consumption of a benzodiazepine for this length of time still makes the consumer at risk of withdrawal symptoms. This has only been reported in two studies, and I was an author of both of them, so I can give more exact details (Murphy et al, 1989; Murphy & Tyrer, 1991; Tyrer et al, 1988).

I apologise for some of the technical language in the following accounts. In the first study, patients were randomly assigned to a flexible dose regime of one to four capsules a day of buspirone (5 mg) or diazepam (5 mg) using a double-blind procedure (neither the patient nor the doctor knew which drug was in the tablets because all the tablets were identical). Half of the patients took active drug for six weeks and then switched abruptly to placebo capsules of identical appearance for the remaining eight weeks of the study, while the other half received active medication for 12 weeks before switching at the end of the study to placebo for two weeks. Thus all patients were taking the capsules over the 12-week period. The patients were given the option of taking up to four capsules daily, but very few did so. The dosage varied between 1.5 and 2.3 capsules daily (i.e. 7.5 to 11.5 mg of diazepam or buspirone).

Figure 7.1 shows the study results in graphical form. The control drug, buspirone, showed some improvement over the 14-week period and did not show the same fluctuations as diazepam. In those taking diazepam, there were brief peaks of withdrawal symptoms at eight weeks in the early-withdrawal group and at 14 weeks after late withdrawal. But you will also notice the increase in symptoms in the early-withdrawal group happened between four and six weeks, when tolerance would have developed to the drug.

In the second study (Tyrer et al., 1988), 210 patients with anxiety and depressive disorders were randomly allocated to five different treatments, one of which was diazepam, and given instructions to reduce all treatments after six weeks so they were completely stopped at 10 weeks. In this study, diazepam was the least effective treatment; it had the worst outcomes by the end of 10 weeks, although not in the initial phase of the study. As there were no assessments between six and 10 weeks, the nature and extent of any withdrawal symptoms could not be shown. These findings (Figure 7.2) show that regular treatment with diazepam for six weeks followed by gradual reduction is clearly associated with withdrawal symptoms and is not beneficial.

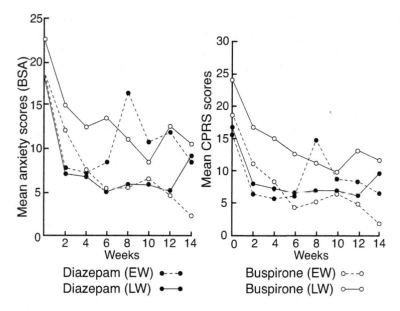

Figure 7.1 Mean score on the BSA and CPRS following early withdrawal (EW) at 6 weeks and late withdrawal (LW) at 12 weeks. The group that took diazepam between 4 and 6 weeks and withdrew early had a two-point increase in the BSA score and a one-point increase in the CPRS score, even before the big jump in withdrawal symptoms at 6 to 8 weeks. Patients who took buspirone did not show this change. BSA = Brief Anxiety Scale, CPRS = Comprehensive Psychopathological Rating Scale. (Reproduced from Murphy et al. (1989) with permission from the British Journal of Psychiatry.)

IT IS WELL KNOWN THAT BENZODIAZEPINES LOSE THEIR EFFECTIVENESS WHEN TAKEN REPEATEDLY

If your work only involves getting people to reduce and ultimately withdraw from taking benzodiazepines, then this statement appears to be true. Those who try to withdraw have often had problems with their medication from the beginning, and when withdrawal symptoms get in the way, any benefits the drug may have had are lodged in the distant past. The tolerance and addiction view can then take over. The suggestion that the only benefit achieved in repeated dosage is by dosage increase seems to be a strong one.

But every doctor who has given prescriptions for benzodiazepines or antidepressants repeatedly knows that this is not true. Only a very small minority of patients increase their dosage, often quite rapidly, and become addicted, often looking for faster-acting drugs and taking them by injection. The others, well over 90% of the total, take their drugs

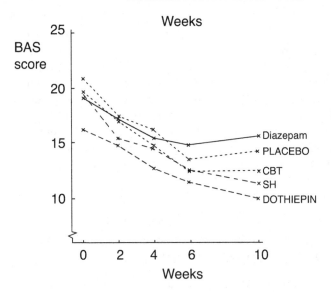

Figure 7.2 Anxiety (BSA) scores for 210 patients randomly allocated to four treatments for 6 weeks followed by withdrawal of treatment over 4 weeks.

as prescribed, always careful not to exceed the dose, and maintain this for many years (Rosenqvist et al., 2023). The Z-drugs have a greater tendency for dosage increase. Patients who take these generally do not have withdrawal reactions and seem surprised that others do. This does not mean that the drugs are necessarily providing a satisfactory response to symptoms, but clearly the tolerance argument is wrong.

IT IS WELL KNOWN THAT BENZODIAZEPINES CAUSE PERMANENT PROBLEMS WITH CONCENTRATION, LEARNING AND MEMORY AND LEAD TO BRAIN DAMAGE

This is also likely to be false, although research in the area continues. In one study (Lader et al., 1984), computer scans of the brain showed loss of brain tissue (atrophy), leading to larger spaces in the ventricles, in patients who had taken benzodiazepines. This was supported by another paper showing memory impairment in long-term benzodiazepine users (Golombok et al., 1988), but these results could not be repeated, and a larger study found no brain abnormality in such patients (Busto et al., 2000). There was unnecessary controversy surrounding the original study as it was suggested that further research had been suppressed by the Medical Research

Council, leading to banner headlines – 'MPs and campaigners predict class action after failures to mount full-scale research into warnings left millions of patients at risk' – but the Medical Research Council did not pursue this area of research after it was not supported by their external assessors.

It has also been suggested that benzodiazepine consumption leads to dementia (He et al., 2019). This again has not been backed up by other good evidence; a much larger nationwide study showed no evidence for any link with dementia. One of the interesting findings was that those who took the drugs in regular higher dosage seemed to have a lower incidence of dementia (Osler & Jørgensen, 2020), so the drugs may have preventive value.

IT IS WELL KNOWN THAT LONG-TERM BENZODIAZEPINE USE MAY AGGRAVATE ANXIETY DISORDERS AND MAKE THEM WORSE

Both the Ashton Manual and numerous commentators make this assertion without any evidence. It is difficult to get really good evidence here; it is not sufficient to point to individual patients who are apparently worse off than they were previously as many factors could be behind the change. The benzodiazepine-dependent patient is not like a gambler who has become destitute after gambling all with no return: such a person cannot point to anything else apart from gambling for their predicament. It is possible to carry out a study that compares the symptoms of patients continuing benzodiazepines after long-term therapy with a similar group of anxious patients receiving, for example, relaxation therapy, to see if the benzodiazepine consumers had more symptoms, but this has not been done. In a long-term study of patients treated with CBT for panic disorder (Brown & Barlow, 1995), those who took additional benzodiazepines had worse outcomes, but this may have just reflected that they were a population with more initial symptoms. The selective experience of patients in withdrawal studies is relevant here. There are many patients who have taken benzodiazepines long term and quietly continue their lives without complaint or changes in their symptoms.

IT IS WELL KNOWN THAT BENZODIAZEPINES CREATE HORRIBLE WITHDRAWAL SIDE EFFECTS WHICH ARE VERY SIMILAR TO COMING OFF HEROIN OR COCAINE

This is often said by those who have never taken heroin or cocaine that the withdrawal symptoms of benzodiazepines are so much worse. The evidence here is more complicated. Withdrawal symptoms from heroin can be severe but usually last for only a week, whereas benzodiazepine drugs have withdrawal problems over a much longer period. But the comparison is unfair; heroin is a highly addictive drug that raises mood and leads to craving and continued use, often in greater dosage, for its pleasure-inducing properties. Benzodiazepines in normal dosage do not create actual pleasure unless you regard the reduction of anxiety as pleasurable. Quite simply, heroin and diazepam cannot be put into the same addiction basket.

IT IS WELL KNOWN THAT EACH PERSON'S EXPERIENCE OF WITHDRAWAL IS UNIQUE

This statement is made in the Ashton Manual (Chapter 2) and is right in one sense but wrong in another. It is right to say that there is great variation in the manifestation of withdrawal symptoms from patient to patient so an individual's pathway through reduction cannot be standardized in any way. Where it is wrong is giving credence to every symptom experienced as a true withdrawal effect. If I attribute every single unpleasant feeling, whether it be a symptom such as tingling in my fingers or stomach churning, a thought such as one of impending doom or a behaviour such as restlessness, to benzodiazepine withdrawal, I leave nothing to other causes. My own psyche and its difficulties are excluded from consideration, and what I had for breakfast is utterly ignored.

The other danger of this universal attribution to withdrawal is the failure to take any personal responsibility for your symptoms or feelings. There is something satisfying in blaming everything that has gone wrong on an external factor that has nothing to do with you. You can afford to sit back and rant against the rash decision of a doctor to treat you with a benzodiazepine and transfer all your rage with impunity: 'I have no responsibility for my terrible state. It is all a consequence of other's incompetence.' This is not the way Heather Ashton is wanting you to think. In the Ashton Manual, she is encouraging all to take responsibility for their own withdrawal regimes and not to rely on others.

IT IS WELL KNOWN THAT 50%–80% OF PEOPLE WHO HAVE TAKEN BENZODIAZEPINES CONTINUALLY FOR A FEW WEEKS OR LONGER WILL EXPERIENCE WITHDRAWAL SYMPTOMS WHEN REDUCING THE DOSE

The proportion of patients who develop withdrawal problems is relatively easy to investigate. I showed this earlier in this chapter. Randomized trials comparing benzodiazepines with other drugs of no dependence potential can demonstrate differences but do not actually give percentages as the data are averages of the group. The proportion with withdrawal symptoms has to be examined by looking at the individual data. In looking at all the data from studies in which these proportions are given, the range extends from 20% to 44%, no matter how withdrawal is defined, even if it is only shown for a few days. But in many of these cases, withdrawal was abrupt; when the withdrawal is gradual, there are generally fewer withdrawal symptoms (Vikander et al., 2010). Nowhere are there any data showing that 50%–80% of otherwise unselected patients have withdrawal problems.

IT IS WELL KNOWN THAT PATIENTS CAN EXPERIENCE HUNDREDS OF WITHDRAWAL SYMPTOMS

The particular difficulty in deciding what exactly defines a withdrawal symptom is discussed in the next chapter. If it is defined as any symptom arising during the withdrawal period, the list becomes very long. Benzo. org.uk gives more than 100 symptoms of withdrawal. It is impossible to decide which of these are true withdrawal effects, which are a return to previous anxiety symptoms, or which are completely unrelated and wrongly attributed to withdrawal by the patient. There are fewer than 20 standard questionnaires developed for the recording of symptoms.

IT IS WELL KNOWN THAT DOCTORS WHO PRESCRIBE BENZODIAZEPINES ARE DRUG COMPANY HACKS

This view is not held in such a bald form by most people but is still shared in some form by many. It is true that there was a time in the past when drug companies were able to court doctors with gifts and free attendance at attractive overseas venues, but this has now been frowned on by all organizations and it is now less common.

In pointing out these errors, I must be fair in reporting many very good elements of the Ashton Manual and the advice of the activist groups like the Benzodiazepine Consortium. Statements such as 'Many "withdrawal symptoms" are simply due to fear of withdrawal (or even fear of that fear)', 'you can reassure your doctor that you intend to be in charge of your own program and will proceed at whatever pace you find comfortable' and 'benzodiazepines occasionally cause paradoxical excitement with increased anxiety, insomnia, nightmares, hallucinations at the onset of sleep, irritability, hyperactive or aggressive behaviour, and exacerbation of seizures in epileptics', are all correct but it is fair to add that the paradoxical symptoms are fairly rare. It is also helpful that most organisations give details of the dose equivalents for each benzodiazepine and which have short or long half-lives.

The paradoxical symptoms (i.e. those that are the opposite of anxiety relief) have to be taken notice of as they are potentially very serious (and are therefore described in the full list of prescribed drugs, the British National Formulary). These symptoms can also be found with antidepressant withdrawal. They can occur independent of withdrawal or during withdrawal and are impossible to predict. As might be expected, those who are involved in antisocial or similar acts and have been taking benzodiazepines or antidepressants often use these paradoxical reactions in their defence; it is very difficult to elucidate the truth in these cases.

In a good prescriber–patient relationship, the competing requirements of the clinic doctor have to be appreciated. If a patient with persistent distressing anxiety comes to the clinic, the doctor does not ask, 'which drug company am I supporting today?' but instead, 'the patient is very upset and suffering quite a bit; what can I do at this point to relieve symptoms?' It is not necessary to prescribe a benzodiazepine, but the doctor knows that this is the quickest route to relief, so it is taken for this reason; it has nothing to do with the demands of others. So some sympathy needs to be shown, and the blame that is heaped on a doctor for starting a patient on a switchback track of pain and withdrawal should be regarded as not completely justified.

GENERAL ADVICE ABOUT STARTING AND STOPPING BENZODIAZEPINES

There have been few voices supporting the continued use of benzodiazepines in the last 30 years, with the important exception of many practitioners who have continued to prescribe them despite all the fuss. When Malcolm Lader (2011) wrote in horror at their high level of continued prescription in an article titled 'Benzodiazepines revisited: will we ever learn?' he was suggesting that only legal threats would bring the profession to its senses. But the experts who disagreed with all the banner warnings decided it was time to fight back. An influential group from the Royal College of Psychiatrists and the British Association for Psychopharmacology reviewed the subject and concluded,

> *Whenever benzodiazepines are prescribed, the potential for dependence or other harmful effects must be considered. However, the group also believes that the risks of dependence associated with long-term use should be balanced against the benefits that in many cases follow from the short or intermittent use of benzodiazepines and the risk of the underlying conditions for which treatment is being provided.*
>
> (Baldwin et al., 2013)

There have been many benzodiazepines marketed for treating anxiety over the last 50 years – chlordiazepoxide, diazepam, medazepam, bromazepam, oxazepam, clorazepate, clonazepam, clobazam – and as long ago as 1973, I criticised the number available as constituting a benzodiazepine bonanza as so many could not be justified clinically (Tyrer, 1974). Most therapists confine their drug prescriptions of benzodiazepines to two or three compounds at the most. The differences between them are relatively small and largely concern how they are metabolised in the body; Chapter 3 explains the science of pharmacokinetics more fully. To understand this and its relevance to drug action there are two areas of importance. The first is the half-life, the duration of time for half of the drug to leave the bloodstream. This can vary from a few minutes to many hours. The second is whether or not the drug has active metabolites, other drugs that have similar effects to the parent drug.

A drug with a short half-life and no active metabolites will quickly be cleared from the body and lose its effects; one with a long half-life will have effects that persist, including if the drug has active metabolites also. If the active metabolites have a longer half-life than the parent drug, they are also likely to accumulate and so prolong drug action (Table 7.1).

The logical choice of a benzodiazepine is determined by the reason for its prescription. A person who is highly anxious in social situations but not in others is best treated with a drug of short half-life and with no metabolites. At the opposite pole, a chronically anxious patient who is slightly more anxious in the evening than the morning might have a long-acting drug with active metabolites and if necessary supplement this with a lower dose early in the evening. The patient's choice sometimes contradicts this as the pharmacokinetics of a drug does not always predict its effects, and in such instances the right policy is to assume the patient is right, particularly if the desired effects are still maintained after repeated prescription.

There is one excellent piece of advice that I learnt very early on in my career, just at the point when benzodiazepines became widely available. It was 'avoid regular prescription'. If you only take a benzodiazepine once or twice a week, it avoids all the problems of tolerance and dependence. The drug, unless it has a very long half-life, will be out of your body within 72 hours and if you take one later it will have the same effect as the first.

MANAGEMENT OF BENZODIAZEPINE WITHDRAWAL SYNDROME

In December 1980, I was visited at Mapperley Hospital by Richard Lindley, a well-known broadcaster noted particularly for his work with Panorama, a programme that is often first in introducing

Table 7.1 Equivalent Doses of Benzodiazepines

Drug (A or H)	Dose equivalent (mg)	Half-life
Diazepam (A)	10	Short in single dosage, long in repeated dosage
Nitrazepam★	10	Long-acting
Oxazepam	20	Medium-acting
Clonazepam	2	Medium-acting
Alprazolam	0.5	Short-acting
Lormetazepam★	1.5	Medium-acting
Loprazolam★	1	Long-acting
Chlordiazepoxide	20	Long-acting
Temazepam★	10	Short-acting
Lorazepam	1	Short-acting
Zopiclone★	5	Short-acting
Zolpidem★	10	Short-acting
Clobazam	20	Long-acting

★Note that zopiclone and zolpidem are similar but are not benzodiazepines.

Short half-life – up to 6 hours; long half-life – over 100 hours (applies to repeated dosage and active metabolites).

important news before any other TV channel has noticed. He must have been a little puzzled by the venue. Mapperley Hospital, now closed, was founded in 1880 was in its last days as a mental hospital, and Richard must have felt strange walking into the turreted entrance and down the long corridors with peeling paint on their walls and just a faint smell, reminiscent of disinfectant, possibly mixed with mould, everywhere. (It is now the headquarters of the Nottingham Health Care NHS Foundation Trust and although it looks the same from outside, it has a sparkling interior, bright lighting and well-proportioned welcoming rooms.)

Richard had come to see me as it appeared that Panorama might have another scoop in their hands. I had written a paper adumbrating the full publication of a study showing dependence problems with people taking benzodiazepines in normal dosage. In this paper, I wrote,

> in a recently completed study of patients who had taken lorazepam or diazepam regularly in therapeutic dosage for four months or more and who then stopped medication abruptly, 27 per cent of those who completed the study had an unequivocal withdrawal syndrome in that they had typical symptoms of abstinence of short duration which then resolved.

(Tyrer, 1980, p. 577)

Richard wanted to highlight this finding in a programme, but I, as a relatively junior researcher, had always been taught not to go public on any research finding until it had been assessed fully and published. So I demurred, saying it would be premature for Panorama to publicise this finding at this stage, as although it was clearly of public interest, we had to wait a little. (In retrospect, I am not sure my sensitivity was justified as the preliminary findings were already in published form, even if not fully scrutinised.)

So Richard went away empty handed, disappointed but no doubt pleased he would not be climbing back up the hill to Mapperley Top, as it was called, with its brooding mental hospital guarding its ridge. Shortly after this, we published our findings in the *Lancet* (Tyrer et al., 1981), closely followed by Hannes Petursson and Malcolm Lader six months later in the *British Medical Journal* (1981). Then the floodgates opened: benzodiazepine dependence was big media business, and everyone had to get in on the story (MacKinnon & Parker, 1982). It was further highlighted by Esther Rantzen and the team on *That's Life* who extracted stories of people behaving completely out of character, living zombified existences and unable to think straight, showing that what the Rolling Stones had called Mother's Little Helper had morphed into Mother's Brittle Yelper.

A correction was needed, but the alarm was over-stated, and many patients who then stopped their benzodiazepines suddenly had very unpleasant experiences. The reaction was an example of what is called the catastrophe theory, a dramatic shift in behaviour from a small beginning. Just a few people had learnt what I have always recommended, take the drugs when you need them, but not regularly. Virginia Ironside, the famous agony aunt of the media, has always come to sensible solutions earlier than most people, and at this time of searing distress she wrote,

> *I take a milligram now and again if tormented thoughts are keeping me awake. It saves an enormous amount of grief. I meet people looking haggard and they say they have been so worried and can't sleep, and I think, you stupid wallies – take a Valium and it'll all look different in the morning. And you'll stop a pattern developing where you wake up at four in the morning day after day.*

The public reaction to the knowledge that benzodiazepine dependence existed was, as I feared when I saw Richard Lindley, over the top. It created harm in promoting fear, despair and anger and because of the nocebo effect, discussed in detail in the next chapter, exaggerated the symptoms of the benzodiazepine dependence syndrome.

This over-reaction was exported to the United States and other English-speaking countries but not to Europe. My French colleagues have always been very sanguine about the use of benzodiazepines. They are used, sometimes excessively, for *le stress*, but there is much less concern about dependence. I have suggested to them that this represents an under-reaction to a significant problem, but as time has gone on, I am beginning to feel they have the reaction right.

When we found withdrawal symptoms in our first study, they were noticed by patients but none were unduly concerned, and they returned to normal by the end of the study. The furore that followed has muddied the waters so much that it is very difficult to be certain what constitutes dependence and what is just a minor hiccup when patients withdraw from medication. In 1986, I wrote a book for the general public about reducing tranquillizers. It was not a great success as throughout the book I was challenging the reader to be more positive about their attitudes to withdrawal symptoms.

I was being a little harsh in some of my comments. 'The main disadvantage of regarding withdrawal symptoms as due entirely to the drugs you have been taking for so long is the tendency to sit back and be virtuous. "Look at the terrible symptoms", you may cry, "all caused by these drugs"' (Tyrer, 1986, p. 67). I was also giving more blame to the patients than was justified:

> *You sought advice from your doctor in the first place because of nervous symptoms, most of which are probably similar in many respects to your present ones. The medical profession is far from blameless as it should have detected tranquillizer dependence earlier, with benzodiazepines in particular, but it is likely that the doctor who first prescribed your tranquilizers had little or no idea of this risk at that time. Indeed, if you have been taking tranquilizers for more than seven years it is almost certain that you were prescribed tranquilizers in all good faith as a safe alternative to the barbiturates and other similar drugs, to help you avoid the risk of dependence with these older compounds.*
>
> (Tyrer, 1986, p. 68)

The average patient is not to know the ins and outs of the history of tranquillizers and should not be made responsible for the errors of others.

But there is a valid point here. There was a big campaign in the 1970s to reduce the prescription of the old tranquillizers, the barbiturates. A government-supported body called Campaign on the Use and Restriction of Barbiturates, nicely abbreviated to CURB) gave a clear message to practitioners. The campaigning group of doctors estimated that 27,000 people had died using barbiturates between 1959 and 1974 and that prescriptions of these drugs could no longer be justified.

'Modern benzodiazepine drugs such as chlordiazepoxide are just as effective as the barbiturates in their therapeutic action, they have fewer side effects, and their addictive potential is low' trumpeted the *British Medical Journal* in 1975, and doctors dutifully followed suit. But after this big shift in prescribing, the evidence that benzodiazepines were similarly influenced by dependence was regarded almost as an act of pharmaceutical sabotage. Why were we being fooled?

But the cycle continued. 'When will they ever learn?' sang Bob Dylan plaintively; 'not in your lifetime, Bob', came the answer. Just at the time that benzodiazepines were being hammered unmercifully, a new range of antidepressants came on the market, the SSRIs. These were found to have benefits in treating anxiety as well as depression, so another big shift in prescribing occurred with these new drugs with no risk of dependence, unlike these nasty benzodiazepines that got everyone addicted. But the bully beating an old drug when it was down was about to suffer the same fate. Before long there were reports of what were called 'discontinuation syndromes' with these drugs (Haddad, 2001). It took some time before this euphemistic phrase was replaced by its true nature, 'withdrawal symptoms', but the discontinuation label still continues to be used (Gabriel & Sharma, 2017),

There was also considerable concern about a possible link between SSRIs and suicidal behaviour (both suicide attempts and actual suicide). One large study suggested such a link (Fergusson et al., 2005); another contradicted it (Gunnell et al., 2005). There is still no clear answer. The same worry about suicide has also been raised with benzodiazepines (Tournier et al., 2023), but there are few suicides caused by benzodiazepines. One worrying aspect of the treatment of depression with SSRIs is the frequent presence of blunting of emotions (Price et al., 2009). This affects decision making and lead the person to errors in dealing with problems, including attitudes to continuing drug therapy and thoughts of suicide.

Withdrawal from benzodiazepines is not a cut-and-dried process. Heather Ashton is right to suggest that each person develops their own way of going about this and even allows them to have 'holidays' when they stop reducing for a short period. In my book, I suggested both short withdrawal programmes of nine weeks and longer programmes when patients are completely in control of their reduction and no time limit is given (Tyrer, 1986, pp. 41–56).

For both benzodiazepine and antidepressant withdrawal, the key is the gradual reduction of medication irrespective of whether you fear withdrawal symptoms or not. If a benzodiazepine or antidepressant has a short half-life (e.g. alprazolam, lorazepam), withdrawal problems are more likely than with a medium or long half-life, and particular care needs to be taken about the speed of withdrawal, particularly early in reduction. The same applies to antidepressants. Paroxetine has a short half-life and is responsible for more withdrawal problems than fluoxetine, which has a long half-life. Some authorities even recommend switching to fluoxetine if withdrawal from other antidepressants in difficult, and, once stabilised, the fluoxetine can be slowly reduced (Gabriel & Sharma, 2017).

ADDITIONAL HELP TO AID WITHDRAWAL

The general notion of helping patients withdraw from benzodiazepines by adding another drug to offset withdrawal symptoms seems sensible and has led to many other studies. But all of them, whether buspirone (Ashton et al., 1990), dothiepin (now dosulepin) (Tyrer et al., 1996) or progesterone (Schweizer et al., 1995), have failed to show greater success in stopping benzodiazepines when given as supporting treatments. There is very slight evidence that the mood stabiliser, carbamazepin, might be more helpful than others (Denis et al., 2006).

Psychological treatments have also been used widely in the management of benzodiazepine withdrawal but have not fared much better than drug supplements. A recent review found treatments such as motivational interviewing ineffective and the most favoured treatment, CBT, were valuable for up to three months but had lost their effectiveness by six months (Darker et al., 2015). The general conclusion of all these studies is that good, supervised care from a GP is probably better and less disruptive than any additional therapy.

SUMMARY OF THE VALUE OF BENZODIAZEPINES

At this point it is useful to summarise the merits of benzodiazepines rather than dwell on their handicaps:

- Most people who take benzodiazepines or antidepressants do not have any problems with continuing their drugs or stopping them when the time comes.
- Very few patients on regular benzodiazepine or antidepressant medication increase their dosage to levels which are above the therapeutic range.
- Despite many admonishments to stop treating patients with benzodiazepines and antidepressants, both doctors and patients appear to be satisfied with the effects of these drugs and, respectively,

continue to prescribe and consume them. These voices have to be listened to, although it needs sensitive ears to pick them up.

- Although many authorities described benzodiazepines as toxic and dangerous, there is very little evidence that they are a cause of death on their own. This is less true of the antidepressants. But most of the fatalities with these drugs are found when taken in a cocktail of other drugs or alcohol that then leads to death.
- There has been substantially less attention given to the withdrawal problems of antidepressants, but it is reasonable to predict that exactly the same will happen as with benzodiazepines and new drugs will be suggested. If one adopts the motto 'every drug that is effective in treating anxiety is also prone to dependence' you will not go far wrong.
- The importance of underlying personality structure has much to do with the problems of withdrawal of these drugs, but it has not been fully acknowledged.

There is now a groundswell of opinion that benzodiazepines have been unfairly stigmatised and need to make a comeback (Balon et al., 2020). I would like to join this clamour, although not too loudly.

MESSAGES FROM CHAPTER 7

1. Benzodiazepines have been prescribed too liberally in the past, and all were complacent before recognising their dangers, primarily over withdrawal problems.

2. Despite these worries, these drugs remain the most effective in the short-term treatment of anxiety and when taken only when required are safe and free of significant problems.

8

THE CONFUSING WORLD
OF WITHDRAWAL

The words 'withdrawal syndrome' are repeated very often when discussing drug dependence, but they have become muddied by misuse. The natural worry that all patients have been led to believe is that they will not be able to stop taking drugs because they have become addicted. This is a relatively recent concern, As Joanna Moncrieff has described it, 'although many people are advised to take psychiatric drugs for long periods after their immediate problems have subsided, the evidence on which these recommendations are based is flawed. This is because the impact of withdrawal effects on the results of research on long-term treatment has been ignored' (p. 181).

This is partly true, but there are many reasons why withdrawal has become such a bogey word, and some of these bear little resemblance to the drugs concerned. There are at least five types of problem that can occur when reducing or stopping a drug, and the explanations for each are very different. They can also merge into one another, and the combinations can give rise to even more explanations of withdrawal phenomena. Deciding which of these indicate unequivocal evidence of an addictive withdrawal syndrome is a difficult task as so often the natural course of the disorder is interrupted.

WITHDRAWAL TYPE 1 – RETURN OF THE ORIGINAL SYMPTOMS PRIOR TO DRUG TREATMENT

Until the late 1970s, a return to previous pathology was the most common explanation for patients becoming unwell again after stopping drugs. This belief was not unreasonable, even though many believe

DOI: 10.1201/9781032619019-9

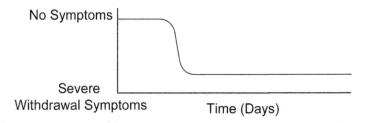

Figure 8.1 Return of original symptoms prior to drug treatment.

it so in hindsight. It is well documented that some mental disorders, especially anxiety, in the absence of treatment, or even with treatment, may continue unchanged for many years (Craske et al., 2017). There was therefore a ready explanation for the reappearance of symptoms after withdrawal. In 'pure' examples of this type of withdrawal problem, the symptoms experienced are exactly the same as they were originally; they are recognised as being the same by the patient and have the same intensity. In such cases, it would be wrong to describe this as a withdrawal symptom.

When I was a practising senior registrar and consultant from 1970 onwards, this explanation of withdrawal problems was by far the most common. The answer, as you might expect, was to suggest to the patient that they return to taking the same dose of drug that they took originally. 'Sorry about this', says the doctor from the past, 'but you clearly need these pills, so here's another prescription'. This may sound odd now, but it is often true, although now in the present climate, with fevered worry about dependence furrowing every brow, it is largely dismissed or ignored.

WITHDRAWAL TYPE 2 – TEMPORARY REBOUND IN SYMPTOMS SOON AFTER STOPPING THE DRUG

A very large number of drugs used for both physical and mental illness suffer from rebound effects after they are stopped (Figure 8.2). Most drugs used for high blood pressure (hypertension) are highly effective and do not lose their potency, but if stopped suddenly, they can lead to a serious rebound in blood pressure. This can be fatal if the heart is put under extra pressure, so the advice is always to withdraw gradually (Koracevic et al., 2021). Propranolol and other drugs called beta-blockers can reduce anxiety in people who have palpitations and other similar symptoms (Tyrer & Lader, 1974), but they also can produce rebound anxiety when suddenly stopped.

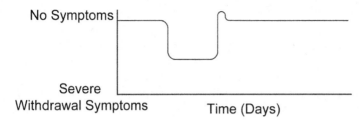

Figure 8.2 Temporary rebound in symptoms after withdrawal.

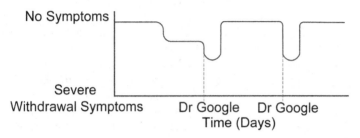

Figure 8.3 The nocebo effect after drug withdrawal.

Rebound anxiety can usually be prevented by gradual withdrawal of the drug concerned. It is usually explained by the sudden uncontrolled return of the normal functions that are suppressed by taking the drug. Gradual withdrawal gives them time to adjust.

In practice, a general rule is advised for patients and prescribers of psychotropic drugs, as well as many other drugs in general medicine: 'always reduce the drug gradually unless there is an unconditional reason for immediate cessation of treatment'.

WITHDRAWAL TYPE 3 – THE NOCEBO EFFECT

The nocebo effect is often forgotten by both prescribers and patients, but it is an important clue to many of the withdrawal problems experienced by patients, so it is discussed in more detail in the next chapter. It is the opposite of the placebo effect ('I will please') as it means 'I will harm' and can influence greatly the outcome of both drug prescription and its withdrawal and is quite independent of drug action: high levels of concern about the dangers of dependence with psychotropic drugs negatively impact the drugs' effects.

To give you a greater understanding of the nocebo effect, I would like to describe a study involving the withdrawal of benzodiazepines in people taking them at normal dose levels. This was carried out in the

1980s, just after the demonstration that low doses of benzodiazepines could cause dependence. In the early 1980s, there was concern about dependence with benzodiazepines but it was not massive, and at that time, the nocebo effect was less than today. The timing is important as it probably influenced the results.

The study sample included patients who had been taking a benzodiazepine for anxiety for six months or longer and wanted help in stopping medication. Those who were on a benzodiazepine that was different from diazepam agreed to change to diazepam in an equivalent dose in advance of withdrawal; diazepam has the advantage of being prescribed in three different strengths, so it can be withdrawn gradually with much greater ease than other drugs. The patients were told that the plan was to have a controlled withdrawal of diazepam in which their medication would be replaced by others of different strengths as part of gradual withdrawal until by the end of three months they would have withdrawn from medication completely. The patients were then randomly allocated to one of two groups in which diazepam was gradually reduced at different times, half reducing early and half later (Table 8.1).

All patients took diazepam in a dose matched to their body weight. In the first two weeks, all patients took the dose that they had taken previously. After this, all the patients thought that they were reducing their drugs gradually, but this was only partly true. In Group 1, the reduction in medication occurred between the second and sixth weeks, after which the patients continued on placebo; in Group 2, the reduction occurred between the seventh and eleventh weeks so that at week 12 all the patients were taking placebo only (Table 8.1).

What were the results? These are shown in Figure 8.4. Overall, patients in Group 1 had an increase in symptoms between the fourth and tenth weeks, and those in Group 2 had this increase between the second and sixth weeks and then a sudden peak in symptoms at 10 weeks. If the symptoms had been a direct result of the actual withdrawal times, there would have been a different pattern (Figure 8.5).

Table 8.1 Design of the Gradual Withdrawal Study

Group	Week 0–2	Week 3–4	Week 5–6	Week 7–8	Week 9–10	Week 11–12	End of Week 12
Group 1	Full dose (D)	½ D, ½ Pl	¼ D ¾ Pl	Pl	Pl	Pl	No drugs
Group 2	Full dose (D)	Full dose (D)	Full dose (D)	Full dose (D)	½ D, ½ Pl	¼ D ¾ Pl	No drugs

Abbreviations: D = Diazepam, Pl = placebo.
Source: Tyrer et al. (1983).

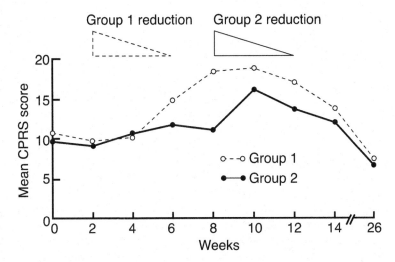

Figure 8.4 Changes in scores on the Comprehensive Psychiatric Rating Scale (CPRS) in Group 1 (early reduction of drugs – dotted line) and Group 2 (late reduction of drugs – solid line). A score of 15 on the CPRS is an indicator of significant symptoms. (Reproduced by permission of *Lancet.*)

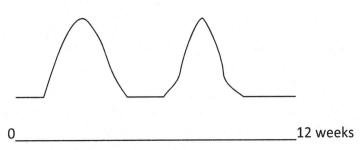

Figure 8.5 Expected results if withdrawal symptoms were linked to dosage reduction.

This design offered the opportunity of recording a range of withdrawal reactions and two forms of nocebo effects (i.e. symptoms occurring at a time when patients thought they were reducing but their drug consumption was unchanged). In the first group, nocebo reactions occurred between the eighth and twelfth weeks when patients were gradually reducing the placebo tablets but thought they were still on a small dose of active medication, and in Group 2, a similar reaction occurred between the second and eighth weeks when patients thought they reducing their medication but in fact were remaining on the same dose.

The actual results can be explained by the nocebo effect. All the patients expected to have a gradual reduction of their drugs after the second week, thinking that the mid-points of withdrawal (8–10 weeks) would probably be the time that their symptoms would be at a maximum. This is what was actually shown in the data (Figure 8.4) except that Group 1, who thought they were reducing immediately after two weeks, had more severe symptoms. The pattern shown in Figure 8.5 did not occur because of the nocebo effect. Patients in both groups experienced apparent withdrawal symptoms when they were not reducing medication, and 41% had pseudo withdrawal or nocebo effects (i.e. withdrawal symptoms occurring when there was no change in drugs).

How does the nocebo effect explain the greater severity of withdrawal symptoms in the early-withdrawal patients in Group 1? Imagine yourself as a patient in the study about to withdraw from your medication at the end of the second week. You are expecting problems, and when they arise soon afterwards, you fear the worst. There is another nine weeks to go, and you expect your symptoms to get steadily worse, so this duly follows. Patients in Group 2 feel differently. They are pleasantly surprised by the absence of withdrawal symptoms at first, and it is only later that they experience them. But now, there are only a few weeks to go, and their expectations are more positive than those in Group 1. As a consequence, their withdrawal problems are not so severe.

This explanation is speculative as we did not question the patients afterwards. Today, this study would probably not pass the scrutiny of a good ethical committee. The element of deception, which you could say is necessary in a study of this nature if you want to examine the nocebo effect, would be unlikely to be countenanced now (Miller & Kaptchuk, 2008), despite the completion of the study with the main aim of withdrawal achieved.

The symptoms experienced in pseudo withdrawal reactions varied (Table 8.2), with some occurring just as frequently as in actual withdrawal. But it should be emphasised that the CPRS is not a specific measure of benzodiazepine withdrawal symptoms, and these are more focused (Tyrer et al., 1990).

A particularly potent form of the nocebo response occurs in many patients who adopt a slow process of withdrawal over many weeks or sometimes months. Heather Ashton, the pharmacologist working in Newcastle mentioned in the previous chapter, worked for many years with patients who had dependence problems with benzodiazepines and developed what is now called the Ashton Manual, in which she warns

Table 8.2 The Most Prominent CPRS Items Separating True Withdrawal from Nocebo Withdrawal Effects

Nature of withdrawal symptom (from CPRS items)	Symptoms occurring during actual withdrawal (%)	Symptoms occurring as nocebo effects (pseudo withdrawal reactions %)
Reduced sleep	30.6★	2.8
Depersonalization	30.6★	2.8
Depression	36.2+	8.3
Reduced appetite	25.0+	2.8
Inability to feel	16.7	16.7
Agitation	16.7	8.3
Hostile feelings	19.4	13.9
Lassitude	16.7	11.1

The top four items (★ P < 0.01, +P < 0.02).

Source: Data taken from Table III in Tyrer et al. (1983).

against coming off benzodiazepines too quickly and often recommends long periods of withdrawal:

> *As a very rough guide, a person taking 40 mg diazepam a day (or its equivalent) might be able to reduce the daily dosage by 2 mg every 1–2 weeks until a dose of 20 mg diazepam a day is reached. This would take 10–20 weeks. From 20 mg diazepam a day, reductions of 1 mg in daily dosage every week or two might be preferable. This would take a further 20–40 weeks, so the total withdrawal might last 30–60 weeks.*

(Ashton, 2002)

Many patients I have seen over the years have adopted the Ashton Manual (many call it a bible as it is so well respected), but it does not explain what I call 'winning post anxiety'. This phenomenon describes the anxiety all tend to feel just when a winning post is in sight: the pressure cricketers are under when there are only a few runs to get yet all the team's wickets are falling, the desperation of football players defending in the last seconds of a game in order to preserve their lead and the leaden feet of the marathon runner who sees the winning post but is now unable to accelerate. The same applies to the person reducing benzodiazepines who has religiously used a sharp knife to split tablets into smaller and smaller doses and is now down to one quarter or one eighth of the tablet, which is the lowest dose prescribed. Stopping this last tablet when the winning post is in sight becomes an almost impossible task. Is this due to

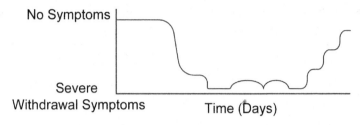

Figure 8.6 Short-term withdrawal syndrome.

the pharmacology of the drug or the psychology of the patient? I think all readers will know the answer (although Horowitz and Taylor [2024] do explain why the reduction is more difficult with lower doses).

WITHDRAWAL TYPE 4 – SHORT-TERM WITHDRAWAL SYNDROME

Most patients who have problems stopping psychotropic drugs have a short-term withdrawal syndrome (Figure 8.6)

Depending on the nature of the drug – benzodiazepines and their analogues usually have problems within a week of withdrawing if they stop their medication suddenly, with a slightly longer delay in those with long half-lives, but antidepressants show their withdrawal problems somewhat later – the course of a short-term withdrawal problem is indicated by an increase in symptoms in the six weeks following reduction followed by gradual reduction. The explanation usually given for this is that the body, more specifically, the receptors in the nervous system, are not able to adjust to the sudden change. Put simply, anxiety generation in the body has been suppressed when taking the drug but when the drug is stopped anxiety returns unopposed. But within a short time, matters are in balance again and the withdrawal problems disappear.

There is not much difference between this type of withdrawal and rebound anxiety. The main difference is one of intensity of symptoms, some of which are new to the patient in this more severe form of rebound. It is a genuine withdrawal syndrome that would not have occurred without previous drug administration.

WITHDRAWAL TYPE 5 – PROTRACTED WITHDRAWAL SYNDROME

The most troubling of withdrawal problems is the protracted withdrawal syndrome (Figure 8.7). This has never been properly explained. If people experience apparent symptoms of withdrawal many years after

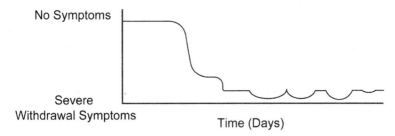

Figure 8.7 Protracted withdrawal syndrome.

stopping medication, it cannot be explained purely by pharmacokinetics as the drug and all its metabolites will have completely left the body. We are left with explanations similar to the 'phantom limb' experiences described in Chapter 3 or other changes, some psychological such as activated memories and some pharmacological in that some long-term changes might been made to receptors in the nervous system that prevent normal balance to be restored.

It is possible, but it would be very hard to prove, that protracted withdrawal is a nocebo response. When I was prescribing benzodiazepines and other drugs in the 1970s, I was not aware of any patients who had prolonged symptoms after stopping benzodiazepines. Was I blind to what was going on around me? Had all these patients quietly returned to taking benzodiazepines when they developed symptoms, or was it actually true that the phenomenon did not exist before the alarm bells about dependence were rung? This is impossible to answer, but as all similar scares about drugs die down eventually, if prolonged withdrawal problems no longer appear in the literature or on social media in the future, this would support the nocebo argument. The hypothesis is that when there is heightened concern about any set of symptoms in medicine more people are likely to suffer from these symptoms than when concern is lessened.

If this was indeed the case, it would not in any way deny the suffering created by prolonged withdrawal. Evidence that these symptoms were not pharmacologically related but caused by psychological factors would in no way reduce the impact of these symptoms or make them any less real. But it would offer a different perspective on a subject that remains highly puzzling to science and to date has no obvious explanation.

This chapter shows that the interpretation of withdrawal reactions is complex and often uncertain, not least as many of these withdrawal types do not have the time scale necessary to confirm their nature. If those experiencing the early symptoms of what they think is withdrawal start taking benzodiazepines again, or indeed other medication, the pattern is interrupted, and it is impossible to say which type of withdrawal reaction it is. It is better to describe these all as symptoms occurring during withdrawal rather that ascribing them to types when there is incomplete evidence.

As a final word about the symptoms of withdrawal I quote something from my book I wrote in 1986. I would not use quite such strong language today, but the message is still relevant:

> *The main disadvantage of regarding withdrawal symptoms as due entirely to the drugs you have been taking for so long is the tendency to sit back and be virtuous. 'Look at the terrible symptoms', you may cry, 'all caused by these drugs. The doctor never told me they were addictive, they never should have been prescribed.' This attitude does not help anybody, least of all you.*

(Tyrer, 1986, p. 67)

This is unfair, as it does not acknowledge the exceedingly unpleasant symptoms that many experience after drug withdrawal. But it reinforces the worry that if you blame everything that is wrong with you on somebody else, you are less willing to exercise your own efforts to change them or accommodate their presence by adjusting your own attitudes.

This dichotomous thinking – I am the innocent party, the doctor is to blame – is one of the reasons behind the writing of this book. If the prescribing relationship is viewed as a joint collaborative venture, this type of thinking does not arise. Neither the prescriber nor the patient is blamed; they look for a solution together.

When somebody mentions 'withdrawal syndrome', you must always ask the question, What type of withdrawal syndrome do you mean? There is unlikely to be a definitive answer, but if you cannot get evidence of a clear link between reducing the drug and the onset of clear symptoms, usually different from those previously noted, you can question whether the drugs are a direct cause.

MESSAGES FROM CHAPTER 8

1. Do not be taken in when so-called withdrawal syndrome is described as evidence of some form of addiction. It has many different facets, and addiction is a relatively small element of them.

2. Remember 'nocebo' as much as 'placebo'. We now live in an age when we suspect adverse effects of all kinds when we take new drugs, but we must not assume they are all a direct consequence of the new molecules entering our bodies.

9

DRUG PRESCRIPTION IN YOUNG AND OLDER PEOPLE

The prescription of psychotropic drugs in young people is akin to a politician fighting an election in which winning is a distant dream. The odds are stacked against success, and almost every pledge and decision can be challenged. The argument that the developing child is too precious a being to be suddenly assailed by strange substances is a strong one, even if some of these young people seem only too pleased to test out strange substances themselves without any encouragement.

The ideal way of joining up psychological and drug treatment in most young people is to have working partnerships between the two groups of practitioners. To extend the political analogy, a coalition is the ideal solution, usually with psychological treatment taking the leading role with pharmacology assisting along the way, for short periods in most instances. Unfortunately, polarisation of attitudes is so common that this ideal is not often met. The major consequence of this, especially in poorly resourced services, is that medication becomes the mainstay of treatment by default and often leads to over-prescription and off-label prescriptions, drugs being used for conditions for which they have not been licensed.

ANTIPSYCHOTIC DRUGS

Currently, over-prescription of antipsychotic drugs appears to be prevalent. They are being prescribed twice as often as they were 10 years ago, mainly for autism and bipolar disorder. The incidence of these disorders is also increasing, and it is easy to see how the decision to prescribe drugs may lead the prescriber to justify a diagnosis that was not thought of before.

DOI: 10.1201/9781032619019-10

Currently in the United Kingdom, three antipsychotic drugs are approved for children and young people, aripiprazole for schizophrenia and bipolar disorder, clozapine for schizophrenia if previous treatment ineffective and risperidone for children over 5 with severely aggressive conduct disorder. A recent study (Radojčić et al., 2023) suggests that this recommendation is not being followed as a large proportion of patients treated had diagnoses of autism, non-affective psychosis (i.e. not schizophrenia or bipolar disorder) or anxiety and depression, conditions that are not approved for antipsychotic drug prescription.

In the United States, there has been a dramatic increase in the diagnosis of bipolar disorder in children, an increase of 40-fold from the previous low level 20 years ago. There is considerable controversy over this subject as some claim that the condition was greatly under-diagnosed in the past. But however the data are interpreted, it does appear that emotional and behavioural problems in children are sometimes diagnosed out of context as a bipolar psychosis (Parry & Levin, 2012). This may partly be a consequence of US psychiatry becoming more biologically focused.

DRUGS FOR ADHD

The prescription of drugs for ADHD is well established clinically but remains controversial, with a vocal minority of psychiatrists arguing that the diagnosis and its treatment are tautological (each justifies the other without any independent confirmation) (Timimi, 2017). There has certainly been a dramatic increase in the diagnosis of ADHD that is hard to explain by greater recognition alone. The availability of drugs such as guanfacine and atomoxetine, both non-stimulant drugs, may also have shifted diagnostic practice as some are troubled by the potential hazards of the amphetamines. One problem that has attracted considerable concern is the effect of regular dosage of stimulants on height. There have long been predictions that adult height may be lower in those taking stimulant drugs and this appears to have been confirmed (Wojnowski et al., 2022) although the difference is not great.

DRUGS FOR ANXIETY AND DEPRESSION

The most recommended drugs for anxiety and depression in children are the SSRIs (Patel et al., 2018), where concern over withdrawal problems is less than in adults. Although the results of trials are relatively positive, the chance opportunity to compare both unpublished and published trial data showed that when the two were combined there was no superiority of the SSRI drugs (Whittington et al., 2004). It is always difficult to be fully confident in the results of drug trials that are carried out by pharmaceutical companies as naturally they will tend to allow only the positive ones to go forward to publication.

Added to this is the relative difficulty of carrying out trials in this population, so good data with large numbers are relatively rare. The changes that have taken place in recent years mirror the experiences in adult populations. Antidepressant use has increased, and the prescription of anti-anxiety drugs such as the benzodiazepines have reduced as concern about dependence has grown (Cybulski et al., 2022). Prescribing trends also show that in deprived communities, prescription is much lower despite the incidence of anxiety disorders being higher, which unfortunately reflects a universal trend (Tudor Hart, 1971). One positive aspect of prescriptions is that although diazepam was very commonly prescribed, prescriptions were rarely repeated (Cybulski et al., 2022). I hope this was a consequence of the policy of taking drugs when required and only if considered necessary.

These data were obtained before the COVID-19 pandemic. There is now growing evidence that mental health problems, mainly anxiety and depression, increased during lockdown and consequent educational disruption (Singh et al., 2020; Theberath et al., 2022), so patterns of prescription may have changed. It is too early to say what the long-term impact will be.

DECISION TO INITIATE DRUG TREATMENT IN YOUNG PEOPLE

Although the decision to prescribe is finally made by paediatricians, psychiatrists or other doctors, a great deal of the pressure both to consult and prescribe comes from others. Parents prefer to choose psychotherapy for their children but are increasingly positive about drug therapy, mainly because of its speed of action. Schools are also responsible for pressure to prescribe drugs as behavioural disturbance in children at school is becoming less tolerated and more medicalized (Al-Haidar, 2008). Prescribers need to be aware of these outside pressures before deciding to prescribe psychotropic drugs. There is a trend to prescribe SSRIs more often in adolescents (Brijnath et al., 2017), and the outcome of these interventions needs to be monitored and any untoward effects noted.

PSYCHOTROPIC DRUGS IN OLDER PEOPLE AND IN THOSE WITH INTELLECTUAL DISABILITY

Older people are more sensitive to the adverse effects of drugs and also are slower to metabolize drugs, so repeated prescription tends to lead to greater accumulation than in younger people. For this reason, the starting dose and maximum dosage are set at lower levels for older people. As most drugs are eliminated from the body by the liver or kidney many compounds are prohibited if there is known liver or kidney disease. As older people are more likely to be taking more than one drug for medical conditions, it is important to check on potential interactions when a psychotropic drug is prescribed. Warnings of such interactions should always be given; most of them are given in the leaflets given with drug prescriptions (even though they are often written in vanishingly small text).

This book is written in an attempt to improve the relationship between prescriber and patient. I have chosen not to include drugs for the treatment of dementia or to write about drugs in those with intellectual disability as in these populations, the decision to prescribe rarely involves the patient. These subjects are discussed in full elsewhere in intellectual disability literature (Bhaumik et al., 2015), and the dramatic developments in dementia treatment are best followed by looking at the Alzheimer's disease website. In addition to donazepil, galantamine, memantine and rivastigmine, there are new drugs waiting to be approved: lecanemab, donanemab and remternetug. While none of these reverse the dementing process, they are increasingly effective at slowing it down.

MESSAGES FROM CHAPTER 9

1. Psychotropic drug treatment in children is increasing. It is very difficult to know if this is a consequence of better recognition of mental health problems or unnecessary over-prescription.

2. Much more care needs to be made when prescribing for older people because of their greater sensitivity to adverse effects and potential interactions with other drugs.

10

UNDERSTANDING THE PLACEBO RESPONSE

There are many references to the 'powerful placebo' in the literature. I would prefer to call it the 'mischievous placebo' because it is so unpredictable and always seems to be playing tricks on us. At times it is powerful, at other times deceiving and, many many times, just plain cheeky.

My own experiences with placebos continue to surprise me. After our first study in 1983, we had a large number of placebo tablets left over. I asked our hospital pharmacy to put them into bottles each containing 28 and to label them 'Dr Tyrer's special tablets'. They did this, and at appropriate times subsequently, I dispensed these at my clinics. Please remember, this was a time when most patients expected to receive a prescription when they saw a doctor, and I dispensed my special tablets when I was not convinced any medication was justified yet felt something extra needed to be given to the consultation.

My special tablets were an outstanding success. Patients were enormously pleased with their effects; some were happy to discontinue them, but others asked for more. The absence of any serious side effects was especially noted. But after a few weeks, I got a message from the pharmacy saying that they had checked with the Pharmaceutical Society and had been advised that they were breaking rules by not indicating the nature of the drug in my special bottles. They said they could relabel them 'Dr Tyrer's placebo tablets' but I decided, possibly wrongly, that this would immediately remove the beneficial effects.

The second placebo experience was another clinical trial, published in 2008. This paper was focused on the management of challenging behaviour in people with intellectual difficulty. This trial also involved a placebo comparison, and placebo actually performed better than the active drugs in this study (Tyrer et al., 2008); again we had spare tablets

DOI: 10.1201/9781032619019-11

at the end of the study. One of the patients who had been randomized to placebo had fared particularly well in the trial and asked to continue on her tablets. After debate, this was agreed to, even though the patient and all the staff treating her knew the tablets were placebos. She continued on these for several months until the supply ran out. For the two weeks afterwards, she suffered some withdrawal symptoms of increased anxiety and irritability. These were regarded by the patient, who had borderline intellectual disability and was fully in tune with the procedure, as withdrawal symptoms even though the staff on the unit said these symptoms could not happen after stopping placebo tablets.

These accounts, and there are dozens more that others could tell, show the ability of placebo in a single pill to create major change. But the breadth of the placebo effect covers so much more than the simulation created by a drug. It also includes many aspects of interactions between patients and therapists that are at the heart of this book. We need to realise that placebos in all forms can generate the same change mechanisms as those that are created by drugs, so much that Colloca and Benedetti (2005) argue that psychosocial and pharmacodynamic effects can be similar, if not identical. So an interview between a patient and a doctor can include no active treatment but still be beneficial by giving the impression of giving treatment when none is present, reinforcing positive past memories, making suggestions that only imply therapeutic content and generally conditioning the patient into a positive frame of mind.

I am sure that many of the readers of this section will have been at an interview, whether it be with a doctor, an employer or another in authority, and found afterwards that you felt so much better, but when you reflect on it, you cannot understand why. The placebo effect of the interview is at work, and your nervous system changes, too. Your brain secretes endorphins, natural opiate-like substances that give you pleasure and a greater sense of well-being. Endorphins also reduce pain and are secreted in large amounts in acupuncture and electro-acupuncture (Han, 2004) so that operations can take place without the need for anaesthetics.

But the acupuncture effects can be created in many other ways; in one large study (Haake et al., 2007), sham acupuncture and real acupuncture produced similar benefits for low-back pain after six months, and these were twice as high as standard physiotherapy treatment. The greatest degree of placebo response in one study of pain was found when patients who were highly suggestible were told that the 'drug' they were taking was quite marvellous and highly effective (De Pascalis et al., 2002). The experimenter was fooling them, but that did not matter; their pain was genuinely reduced without any painkiller being present.

How is this relevant to drug treatment for mental illness? In 2008, Irving Kirsch and his colleagues analysed data from 47 clinical trials of depression (Kirsch et al., 2008). They found that in mild depression, placebo was as effective as antidepressants, and it was only in severe depression that relatively small differences in favour of the antidepressant were found. The study was both criticized by pharmacologists and praised by the drug-centered lobby, including Joanna Moncrieff and her colleagues, and it is still a big subject of debate. But even supporters of the efficacy of antidepressants accept that the data show prominent placebo responses that have been increasing in size over time (Khin et al., 2011).

THE NOCEBO EFFECT

The nocebo effect is discussed more fully in the next chapter. It is exactly the opposite of the placebo effect. It is the expectation that a prescription of a drug, an interactional event such as an interview, the viewing of a film, the argument on the bus or indeed any other negative confrontation, can make you feel worse (Planés et al., 2016). In controlled studies, again using pain as the outcome, it has been shown that negative verbal suggestions trigger the activation of a substance called cholecystokinin. This hormone comes from the gut and helps to stimulate digestion, but it also induces anxiety and promotes pain in higher amounts (Benedetti et al., 2007).

IMPLICATIONS OF THE PLACEBO AND NOCEBO RESPONSE IN THE PATIENT–PRESCRIBER PARTNERSHIP

Placebo and nocebo effects can be shown in several ways in the course of a clinical interview for a prescription and its consequences. If the prescriber is respected, and subsequently liked, by the patient, there will be an immediate placebo effect. But it has other consequences. The trouble with the sentiment 'I like this doctor, and I trust them, and am sure whatever is prescribed will be right for me' is that this is exactly the same response that the experienced snake oil seller creates, but the snake oil product is almost certainly completely useless. That is, although a placebo response at the interview has clear advantages, not least that the patient is likely to follow the advice given, it carries negative connotations too. If the charming doctor says at interview, 'I am going to prescribe drug X for you; it always works in your condition', it will also promote the placebo response to the drug. The drug may confer no beneficial properties – a true placebo – but when the patient reports back at the next interview, both feel they have chosen a winner.

It is often said that a placebo effect is temporary, but if it is being reinforced, it can last for years. My patient who continued taking placebo tablets after our clinical trial was convinced the tablets were helping her. So every time she took a tablet, this belief was reinforced, as was the nocebo effect when she eventually ran out of tablets.

The nocebo response at an interview is even more damaging. Even if the advice is sound, the prescription perfectly appropriate and the manner and duration of the drug's effects accurate, the patient will be annoyed, be more likely to reject the advice and may not adhere to the drug correctly. It may sound odd, but the content of an interview to discuss the prescription of a drug has the same power of success or failure as the actual drug itself; a good interview doubles the chance of a successful outcome in drug therapy, an advantage that should not be missed.

MESSAGES FROM CHAPTER 10

1. The placebo response is a highly important part of treatment with a psychiatric drug. It begins with the clinical interview.

2. The nocebo response is just as strong as the placebo one and can be mainly responsible for the failure of an effective drug.

11

DEPRESCRIBING

There is a tendency for people to take more drugs for both physical and mental disorders as they get older. This is not surprising as illnesses become more frequent with advancing age. Sometimes the number and frequency of drugs becomes excessive, and when this combination involves many drugs, it is described as polypharmacy.

It is not surprising that prescribers and drug monitoring bodies have been paying more attention to polypharmacy and feel it should be reduced whenever it is shown to be unnecessary. This has been the stimulus behind what is called deprescribing but could equally be called rational prescribing, the sensible use of drugs. Officially, deprescribing is a structured approach to identifying and discontinuing medications when existing or potential harms outweigh existing or potential benefits. There is another aspect of the subject not in the definition and that is cost: unnecessary drugs lead to unnecessary additional costs.

This book attempts to improve the relationship between prescriber and patient by establishing drug prescription as a joint partnership. The growth of deprescribing is a good illustration that this partnership is failing: the decisions made in deprescribing tend to be unilateral; they are made by professionals who identify unnecessary combinations of drugs and replace them with simpler ones that are just as, or more, effective. But if a good partnership had existed before polypharmacy, the unnecessary prescriptions would not have been given.

It is perhaps not surprising that so many of the studies on deprescribing are concerned with populations in which joint partnership is either difficult or not possible for a number of reasons. There is a special difficulty with clinical populations in intellectual disability and dementia, where polypharmacy is particularly common (Adams et al., 2023; Mueller et al., 2018), and with patients whose voices are very

DOI: 10.1201/9781032619019-12

quiet if not silent altogether. In one recent study, 40% of all patients with dementia were taking four drugs or more daily (Mueller et al., 2018), and those taking more drugs were more likely to be hospitalized, although this is not necessarily a cause-and-effect relationship.

Sawan et al. (2021) are critical of most studies as they are

> limited in scope as most studies focused on medication-related outcomes (e.g. discontinuation of high-risk medications) rather than patient-centered outcomes in individuals living with dementia. Furthermore, most studies focused on addressing inappropriate polypharmacy in older adults with dementia living in long-term care facilities, and interventions did not involve the person and their carer. Further evidence on the impact of deprescribing in this population across clinical settings is needed.

Put more bluntly and in less words, polypharmacy without clinical outcome measures indicates nothing.

Good deprescribing should be a joint exercise. Outside experts should not unilaterally decide that drugs are no longer necessary; some patient involvement is needed, or in the case of dementia, appropriate carers. At present, deprescribing is set up rather like a criminal trial. An offence has been committed – the excessive use of drugs – the prosecution case is heard with very little time spent on any arguments for the defence and the verdict is always guilty as the defence has very little opportunity to argue its case, if at all.

There is more to deprescribing than simple reduction of drugs, even though the literature would suggest otherwise. Most published studies are narrative accounts of what happens during withdrawal, and very few are set up as controlled trials linked to outcome. There are four elements involved in deprescribing, and all are worth examining independently.

UNNECESSARILY HIGH DOSAGE

This is part of deprescribing, but it really refers to reduced prescribing, not necessarily stopping the drug entirely. Patients are in a very good position to identify this element. If a patient is taking a drug for long enough to become familiar with its effects, both beneficial and negative, the need for reducing the drug becomes apparent when it either no longer seems to be of benefit or creates much more severe side effects than it did previously. The evidence of lack of benefit often comes through error, such as when a person goes on holiday and forgets to bring a supply or fails to get a new prescription when one is due but notices no ill effects. Additionally, if side effects become more severe, then patients will tend to reduce their dosage accordingly and often suffer no ill effects; in these cases, the deprescribing is carried out by the patient before it becomes formalized by the prescriber. Meanwhile, unnecessary prescription is followed by unnecessary consumption.

UNNECESSARY POLYPHARMACY

Many patients, probably far too many, take an excessive number of differently named psychotropic drugs, but more enquiry is needed to separate sensible from unnecessary polypharmacy. The latter is particularly frequent in the elderly, where at any one time both prescriber and patient are juggling with different dosages to reduce the risk of adverse effects, drug interactions and changes in symptoms (von Buedingen et al., 2018). The combined use of hypnotic and anti-anxiety drugs is particularly frequent. This form of inappropriate polypharmacy was found in nearly half of all patients referred to psychiatric services in the 1970s (Tyrer, 1978) but is bound to be less today with the somewhat reduced prescription of benzodiazepines.

In many of these instances, the motto seems to be 'playing safe', deciding not to reduce or stop a drug as the patient is satisfied even though the drug may no longer be needed. In a system where repeat prescriptions are often given without any thought, it is necessary every so often to sit back and see if each of these drugs is justified. This initiative can be instigated by the GP, the patient or by local pharmacists, who are becoming much more active in monitoring drug prescriptions (Paloupi et al., 2023). They have even been proposed as polypharmacy stewards whose task would be to monitor all prescriptions (Daunt et al., 2023). An excellent example of a partnership between patient and prescriber would be an annual joint check for all those taking two or more psychotropic drugs where personal and professional views are usefully joined.

LONG-TERM DRUGS PERCEIVED
AS NO LONGER NEEDED

The important word in the title of this section is 'perceived'. This can be interpreted in different ways, but at its core is the patient's perception. If the patient feels that a drug is still helping his or her symptoms, this has to be respected. The wish can be part of the playing safe policy mentioned in the previous section, but it should not be dismissed on that score alone. There can be occasions when the drug has to be reduced or stopped, for example when a new drug has to be given that interacts potentially dangerously with one already being taken; then there is no choice.

When there is doubt about the reduction of a drug, the best policy is to have a short period on a lower dose before making any long-term decisions. This depends to some extent on the drug being reduced. In the case of psychosis, both bipolar and schizophrenic forms, it is always wise to be aware that relapse may be delayed. Stopping drugs with marked side effects after many years of use seemed to appear reasonable (Murray et al., 2016), but it has now been shown that over the long term, in most cases of first-episode schizophrenia, relapse will occur at some point and also lead to early death (Tilhonen et al., 2018).

With these disorders, it is also prudent to be very cautious about dosage reduction unless the patient is being greatly troubled by adverse effects, particularly movement disorders such as Parkinsonism and tardive dyskinesia. There is also a short delay before withdrawal effects may be noticed on reduction of antidepressants. But in many cases of polypharmacy, more than one antidepressant is being taken, and in these circumstances, reduction might proceed more rapidly.

The only useful studies of the value of deprescribing are ones in which patients who are not reducing their drugs are compared with those who are. If deprescribing is completely justified, then there would be no differences between the two groups. Such a study, on the deprescribing of antidepressants, was recently completed in the United Kingdom and published in the *New England Journal of Medicine*, a top-rated medicine journal. In this study, 478 patients in 150 general practices who had a history of at least two episodes of depression in the past or had been taking antidepressants continuously (citalopram, fluoxetine, sertraline or mirtazapine) for two years or longer were recruited to the study if they felt it was an opportune time to stop their antidepressants. Two years of continuous dosage could be regarded as unnecessary as depression is an episodic condition.

The patients were randomized in a controlled trial with half continuing on their antidepressants (maintenance group), and the other half reducing slowly with the help of matching placebos (discontinuation group) (i.e., the deprescribing one) with the reduction programme being similar to the design of the 1986 study described in the previous chapter. After a period of one year, relapse (measured as another depressive episode) occurred in 92 of the 238 patients (39%) in the maintenance group and in 135 of 240 (56%) in the discontinuation group, a highly significant difference indicating greater relapse in the discontinuation group.

The trial is described in bald and uncontentious prose, as is appropriate for a sensitive subject in which opinion always has to be subservient to the science. In the paper, no opinions are given about the implications of the study, and no complaint can be made about this. But there are thousands, if not millions, of people taking long-term antidepressants who are clearly keen to know what the implications are for their medication practice. There were several important clues suggesting what was going on during the 52 weeks of the study, all of which are relevant to deprescribing policy:

1. By the end of the trial, 39% of the patients in the discontinuation group had returned to taking an antidepressant prescribed by their clinician.

2. Quality-of-life measures and symptoms of depression, anxiety, and medication withdrawal were greater in the discontinuation group.

3. A greater percentage of patients in the discontinuation group than in the maintenance group stopped taking the trial medication before the end of the trial (48% vs. 30%).

4. By the end of the trial, 39% of the patients in the discontinuation group had returned to taking an antidepressant prescribed by their clinician, which may explain why there was no evidence of between-group differences for secondary outcomes at the last follow-up at 52 weeks.

   By the end of the trial, 39% of the patients in the discontinuation group had returned to taking a prescribed antidepressant.

Here you can imagine these patients, who constituted an increasing number beginning six weeks after the trial started, saying to themselves, 'I am beginning to get my old symptoms back. I guess I must be in the discontinuation group and this is bothering me. It is becoming clear to me that I still need them. I will persist but if this goes on, I will stop my tablets, which I know are being replaced by dummies, and go back to my doctor.' Taking the definitions of withdrawal described in Chapter 9, these patients are suffering a mixture of rebound symptoms (ones that would improve if they persisted with withdrawal), return to previous symptoms (which the patient might conclude if they stuck it out for a few more weeks but did not get better), nocebo symptoms (the incorrect psychological conclusion, enhanced by worry that they may be getting their old symptoms back) and true withdrawal symptoms (ones that were more severe than expected and lead to an urgent GP appointment to prescribe the antidepressant again). Note that we cannot be sure which of these apply in any individual case because the sequence was interrupted by other drug decisions.

> *Quality-of-life measures and symptoms of depression, anxiety and medication withdrawal were greater in the discontinuation group.*

This tells us quite clearly that the patients in the discontinuation group were not merely disengaging from the trial at a greater rate than the maintenance group through caprice or regret that they were in the trial at all but because they were suffering an increase in symptoms.

> *A greater percentage of patients in the discontinuation group than in the maintenance group stopped taking the trial medication before the end of the trial.*

This confirms the earlier impressions. The patient directly attributed the symptoms to drug withdrawal. As such, the obvious remedy was to stop the tablets irrespective of which group the patient was in. The fact that 92 (39%) of the maintenance group also relapsed during the 12-month trial (they had another depressive episode) represents a mixture of the nocebo effect ('I am sensitive to the presence of new symptoms and think I am getting them so I'm probably in the discontinuation group'), or, as Joanna Moncrieff would predict, these antidepressants are 'not much cop, I told you so'.

> *By the end of the trial, 39% of the patients in the discontinuation group had returned to taking an antidepressant prescribed by their clinician.*

The authors had to explain one of the findings that at first seemed counter-intuitive, that there were no important differences between the groups for a range of secondary outcomes at the final follow-up at 52 weeks. Of course not, as the patients who had bothering symptoms were all back on antidepressants again by the time of the last assessment.

Critics of this trial might point to the troubling fact that of over 23,000 patients considered for the trial, less than 3% satisfied all the needs for randomization. But this would be unfair, as the patients were recruited from many different centres, and bias was essentially removed by the trial design. The merit of the trial is that it shows that deprescribing is a messy business and that those who provide simple solutions are almost always wrong. You cannot predict what is going to happen when a drug is being withdrawn, as the patient, the most important element in the withdrawal, becomes a loose cannon in the process. If all of them had stuck it through the withdrawal regime, we would know which withdrawal subtypes would be manifest, but everybody varies.

The implications of this study for deprescribing policy.

Although the number of patients relapsing was significantly different in the two groups (92 versus 135), it was not dramatic. Although 39% of the patients in the discontinuation group returned to taking antidepressants again, that means that 61% did not. For this 61%, the stopping of antidepressants was presumably beneficial; they no longer needed them. This could then be regarded as successful deprescribing, but for the 39% who went back to taking antidepressants, the case was the opposite: deprescribing had done nothing for them.

We cannot repeat expensive randomized trials to get answers here, but it is relatively easy to record what happens to the drug habits of patients after a deprescribing decision has been made. If almost all of the patients stay off the drugs that have been deprescribed, the enterprise can be regarded as successful. Without such data, deprescribing cannot be assessed satisfactorily.

It would help greatly if there were some way of separating the patients in the big deprescribing trial who stayed off antidepressants and stayed well from those who did not. I would argue, as indeed I have done (rather tediously) in previous parts of this book and elsewhere (Tyrer, 1984, 2010) that understanding the personality of the patient withdrawing from the drug is key to success. In our 1983 study, we found differences in personality features between those who had withdrawal problems and those who had none. These were mainly shown in the traits of dependence, sensitivity and impulsiveness, which when present strongly increased the incidence of withdrawal problems. Personality features of greater passivity and dependence were also shown in the study by Schweizer et al. (1988) during benzodiazepine withdrawal, and similar findings also found by Tönne et al. (1998). Personality status is clearly not going to be the only factor leading to withdrawal or relapse, but it should be addressed.

The best example of personality problems creating significant polypharmacy is emotional instability, or borderline personality disorder. National studies in Europe have shown that only 10% of patients admitted to hospital with borderline personality disorder were not taking a psychotropic drug, with 54% taking three or more, and three quarters taking an anticonvulsant or an antipsychotic drug (Bridler et al., 2015). These are all off-label prescriptions.

Quetiapine was the most common antipsychotic drug, and another study of overdose in those with borderline personality disorder found quetiapine to be the most frequent cause of serious threat to life in two-fifths of all the patients (Ning et al., 2023). The psychology of prescribing unnecessarily in this condition is relevant here. If you have sudden and unpleasant emotional storms, a pill seems to present the best way of managing it, even if it is inappropriate. Fineberg et al. (2019) have novel suggestions about treatment, including greater use of as-required medication for acute episodes, another example of the need for other people around the patient to take an active part in management without the use of drugs.

The greater use of drugs in such personality disorders cannot be ignored. The experience with borderline personality disorder shows, at least to the drug companies, that there is a market in drugs for the condition. Despite these having no clear value in the treatment of this condition (Stoffers-Winterling et al., 2022), I know from recent conversations with others in the United States that many more drug companies are developing products for this market. Inappropriate prescribing is not a reason for them to slacken off here, however it might seem to others.

The *New England Journal of Medicine* trial is described in detail in this chapter as it is probably the only good example of a large controlled trial in which continuation and deprescribing groups can be compared. We need many more of these to separate those symptoms that are definite consequences of reducing or stopping a drug from those that are essentially nocebo reactions. This separation cannot be made from the nature of symptoms alone as the nocebo generated symptoms can be exactly the same as true drug withdrawal symptoms.

CONSENSUS DEPRESCRIBING

I hope this chapter has clarified the most important part of deprescribing, a proper consensus between the patient and prescriber. A prescriber who is determined to get a patient off what appears to be an unnecessary drug will usually fail if the patient is equally determined to stay on it. In today's drug traffic on the Internet, a replacement can always be found. If the patient feels very strongly that continuation is required, a full analysis of the reasons needs to be made, even if the reasons at first seem to be odd, off-beam and pharmacological nonsense. No active pharmacological drug is devoid of adverse effects, and the loss of these may sway the patient towards the deprescribing option.

If deprescribing is decided on by consensus and not forced in any way, then any withdrawal problems are more likely to be overcome without immediately returning to the drug or taking a previously higher dose. This is one of the key elements of nidotherapy: the decision to make changes with full acceptance of the need is manifest in the patient's determination to make the reduction work.

Whatever difficulties are found in the prescriber–patient partnership initially, they can always be overcome without invoking the authority of the time-honoured but now redundant 'doctor knows best' argument or bullying the patient into an essentially one-sided agreement. A sensible, informed and rational drug regime can be achieved with a joint decision that makes the best use of medication and serves the patient well. What more is wanted? Once we have this collaboration, the word 'deprescribing' will be of historical interest only.

MESSAGES FROM CHAPTER 11

1. Deprescribing indicates a failure of good prescriber–patient partnership, as it is usually made unilaterally.

2. Studies of unnecessary psychotropic drug prescription should always be accompanied by follow-up studies of outcomes.

12

PRESCRIBING POLICIES

After a set of chapters helping to set the scene for good prescriber–patient partnerships, we now have to plunge in and show how it can work in practice. Here I will describe four different scenarios between prescriber and patient, and I add the right way of responding to the patient, Maureen, who was described in the introduction to this book.

SCENARIO A: THE FRUSTRATED MUSICIAN

The patient, Charles, is a violin player in a philharmonic orchestra and has become increasingly concerned about errors he is making when playing at major events. He first noticed this when he was very anxious about his four-year-old son, who had developed a high fever, and this was just before a major performance in a different city. His wife persuaded him to go and play and reassured him that she could deal with any eventualities. He did travel, but his anxiety increased as he entered the concert hall. His standards as a violinist were very high, and he always picked up any mistakes. During the performance, he noticed his hands were trembling, and this was clearly affecting his performance, particularly when playing vibrato when he most wanted to show his skills. Although his son quickly recovered, Charles could not forget his poor performance when anxious and feared his next public engagement. To his horror, he found his poor playing repeated, and his anxiety heightened again. After a series of these episodes, he felt he had to consult his doctor.

Doctor: Hello, I'm Dr Brenchwood, I don't think you've consulted here before, although I know your son has been seen by us. Tell me about the problem.

DOI: 10.1201/9781032619019-13

Charles: I feel embarrassed about this as I'm not a nervous person, but I'm a musician, and I'm getting so anxious when I'm playing that it's affecting my performance.

Doctor: What instrument do you play?

Charles: The violin, and normally I'm a pretty good player, but not when I'm anxious.

Doctor: What exactly goes wrong now when you are playing?

Charles: I get progressively more anxious when playing, especially before a solo, and find that my body goes stiff and my hands start to tremble, and, as you might guess, this really gets in the way when playing the violin.

Doctor: So it's the physical symptoms that really bother you, and then your performance suffers.

Charles: That's right, and once I have them, they seem to feed off each other, and my playing gets worse.

Doctor: Are you anxious in other situations? Would you describe yourself as an anxious person, or having an anxious constitution?

Charles: Absolutely not. My wife does tend to get anxious, and she says I will never understand her as I am built so differently.

Doctor: Have you had any treatment for this?

Charles: Nothing of any note. My friends in the orchestra taught me some relaxation exercises and suggested I tried mindfulness before performing, but it did not really help. It's gone on now for over a year and I'm desperate to get rid of it.

Doctor: What type of help were you looking for?

Charles: I just thought there might be a pill I could take, like Valium.

Doctor: There is indeed a pill you can take, but I would not recommend Valium as we would not like you dropping off to sleep during a performance. I'm going to suggest you take a small dose of a drug called propranolol about an hour before you perform, as I think this will help greatly.

Charles: In what way?

Doctor: Propranolol in high doses is prescribed for heart problems. But in low dosage, it reduces trembling and also slows your heart rate a little. It does this by a direct effect on the muscle, not your brain, so you do not get sleepy or have any other side effects like that. But if you suffer from asthma, I would not give you this one but choose another.

Charles: No I do not have asthma; I've no breathing problems. How often do I take it, and for how long?

Doctor: You only need to take it before you are playing in performances. So I will only prescribe you 20 tablets. Each one is 10 mg, and you may find one is enough to take away the tremor, but some people need to take two. How often do you perform in the orchestra?

Charles: I only have a public performance about once every month. I don't have this problem when practising.

Doctor: Good, then 20 tablets will be enough, but I would like to see you in a month's time to see if they are working

If we analyse this conversation, a short one that could be completed in six minutes, we can identify all the elements in good partnership:

- Politeness in introduction and recognition of son's problem
- Focus on the main issue, anxiety when playing the violin
- Probing about the actual problem in practice
- Access (briefly) to the patient's personality structure, finding out that he is not normally anxious
- Enquiry about past treatment with psychological options mentioned, but with a clear message from the patient that he does not want to go down that route
- Nature of prescription explained; important as without it, patient could have left the clinic thinking he had a heart problem
- Frequency of prescription and size of tablets indicated, so patient has a clear indication of when to take the medication

As is readily apparent, since the patient is taking the medication very intermittently, there is no need to discuss the issue of withdrawal. Furthermore, it helps greatly in this example that the patient and doctor understand each other and get on well.

SCENARIO B: THE ANXIOUS PATIENT WITH MANY PAST PROBLEMS

The patient, Mary, is 26 and has a history of physical abuse as a child, a failed marriage followed by divorce and difficulties in her work as a cleaner in a large organisation where she is bullied and subjected to sexist comments by her supervisor. She is seeing a doctor at the same medical centre where she saw a different doctor a month before who put her on diazepam 5 mg twice daily but told her it was unlikely to be repeated as diazepam was addictive.

Doctor: Good morning, I'm Dr Whatten, I don't think we've met before?

Mary: No, it was a different doctor. He gave me a prescription for Valium tablets but said they were addictive, and I could only take them for a short time.

Doctor: Yes, I can see that from the records. But the important thing is how are you now? Are you better than you were before?

Mary: Yes, I am. The new tablets have helped a lot, but as the other doctor said I could only be on them for a short time, I've been trying to come off them in the past week. But I'm not so good without them. I'm not sure what to do. I know that some doctors cross people off their lists if they stay on tablets like these, and I wouldn't like that.

Doctor: Can we just go back a bit. What were the problems that you had when you came a month ago?

Mary: I was just at the end of my tether at work. I was being bullied all the time by Jeff; he's my supervisor, and he was making all these rude comments about my bust and my general appearance. I got so frightened just going into work, so I had to get help.

Doctor: So you just got anxious about the problems at work?

Mary: No, I've always been a worry guts and a whittler. I'm like my mum; she was born nervous and it stuck with her all her life. But things happen to me, I attract trouble, and that makes me more nervous.

Doctor: So if I saw you a year ago, would you have been as nervous as you are now?

Mary: Yes, I suppose so. I would have been very nervous coming to see you.

Doctor: So would it be right to say that you and anxiety have been together all your life as it were, and, if so, what difference have the tablets made?

Mary: For the first time in my life, I felt better; it was like a dark cloud had been lifted from over me. But since I started reducing them, I've been going back to how I was before.

Doctor: The reason you have felt better is that you have been taking a drug that takes away anxiety without knocking you out, as most of the previous drugs did. The main problem with it is that it can cause dependence in some people, and because you have always been an anxious person and had many problems in your life, I think you would become dependent if you continued it regularly.

Mary: So what should I do about it?

Doctor: We have to make a decision now that might be long term. Your type of anxiety is very troubling but not crippling. The official guidance tells us psychological treatments are just as good as drug treatment and it is just a question of which you would prefer. We have two options. The first is continued drug therapy. This would involve continuing to take diazepam, preferably when you feel you require it rather than regularly, and knowing you might become dependent if you take it regularly, or we switch to another drug, one of the antidepressants, as they help in anxiety too. The second is referral for psychotherapy, which can come in several forms, including forms of self-treatment that you can practise at home.

Mary: I just don't know. It's quite a decision. I'm a bit worried about talking to others about my problems as it gets me so uptight, but I suppose there is no risk of dependence then (laughs). What would you recommend?

Doctor: This is really up to you. It could be argued that as you've had such a good response to diazepam it is reasonable to continue this but only when you feel you need it. If you only took it occasionally, there would be no risk of dependence.

Mary: I'll go with that then.

Doctor: Good. Now just to check on how often you might need the tablets, can you keep a diary of when you take it and bring it back to see me in three weeks time?

What were the elements in his conversation that made it a good partnership?

- Good listening. The doctor is giving the opportunity for the patient to express her concerns and carefully deduces the fact that she has an anxious disposition that is part of her personality structure.
- He gives the opportunity for the patient to describe exactly how she felt after taking the diazepam, not just a simple 'has it helped or not?'
- He explains the risk of dependence if Mary continues to take diazepam regularly but does not regard this as a disaster and immediately turn to other drugs which also have dependence risks.
- He gives the opportunity for Mary to decide on whether she shifts to new medication or not. This is the right way of tackling this issue, as there is no clear solution to the choice of drug.
- As Mary turns the question back to the doctor, he makes the decision to continue with diazepam but attempts to make it an as-required drug rather than one taken regularly.
- He tries as hard as possible to get Mary to choose the type of treatment for her anxiety. Her comment about psychotherapy is quite a frequent one. Her impression may be unfair as the

psychological treatment she fears is one that explores every aspect of her past life, which would not be true. But reluctance to talk about yourself to strangers about personal matters is very common, and many people prefer drug treatment for that reason.

SCENARIO C: THE PATIENT WITH A PSYCHOSIS WHO WANTS TO STOP MEDICATION

This scenario must be repeated hundreds of times daily up and down the country. Very few people are pleased with taking antipsychotic drugs. The decision to stop drug treatment is an important one that is usually made by a psychiatrist.

Derek was diagnosed with schizophrenia 20 years ago and has been taking flupenthixol 6 mg daily for the last four years. Before then, because he was suspected of not being reliable about taking his drugs, he had been taking the same drugs by intramuscular injection in a long-acting form, flupenthixol decanoate every month. But he had persuaded his psychiatrist and community mental health nurse that he could be trusted to take his drugs by the oral route, and this had proved successful. But he now felt it was time to stop taking them.

Doctor: Good to see you again. I think your remember me, I'm Dr Mickelover, and your own doctor has just been in touch. He says all has been going well?

Derek: Yes and no. I'm feeling very well apart from side effects from the tablets. I'm putting on weight, and I've been told by my GP that in the prediabetic range, and I can't perform sexually as I would like with my girlfriend. I've thought a lot about it, and I think its time I came of the tablets now.

Doctor: I can quite understand your feelings, and I agree that it's a worry that you might be getting diabetes. But we need to be very careful about stopping your drugs entirely. There is now good research evidence that shows that people with your type of illness are about twice as likely to relapse as those who stay on their drugs, and this is true after many years of treatment before the drugs are stopped.

Derek: Yes, but even if twice as many relapse, it still means that a lot of patients who withdraw stay well.

Doctor: Fair enough, but just remember what it was like when you were last ill and had to be admitted to hospital. I seem to remember you were in for six weeks or so, and it was a long time before you returned to work.

Derek: Can I just try stopping them for a month and see how I am then?

Doctor: That is not much help, I'm afraid. Because the drug effects are still showing in your body after you stop, it is likely that even if you were going to relapse, this would not occur till later.

Derek: What would you recommend then?

Doctor: The main problem seems to be those side effects. They are troubling and serious, and we cannot ignore them. But the positive aspect here is that these side effects in particular depend on dosage. If you take a smaller dose, say 4 mg a day, this may offset the side effects sufficiently to improve your sex life and prevent you from becoming formally diabetic, with all the extra problems that will come along with that diagnosis. Does that seem a reasonable compromise?

Derek: Yes, I think I could go along with that. But if it goes well, I might want to go even further in reduction.

Doctor: We need to take one reduction at a time. And before I write out the new prescription, I want to add something more. You have been very good in sticking to the dose you are on now, but before we put you on oral drugs, you were felt to be unreliable and that's why we chose the long-acting injections. But if I was in your shoes now, and keen to be off the drugs altogether, I might be tempted to ignore the advice I am giving and reduce much more rapidly. All I am asking you to do is to be honest about the drug dose you actually take. If you reduce too rapidly and relapse, you will be in for a difficult time. If you reduce slowly, as I suggest, and then have a relapse, it is likely to be a milder and shorter relapse that we could deal with without hospitalisation.

Derek: What are the chances of relapse when I reduce to 4 mg a day?

Doctor: I would really be guessing in the long term. But in the short-term, up to six months, I would say odds of four to one against.

Derek: Thanks for that. I'll think of it when I bet on a four to one favourite at my next race meeting.

In addressing this common problem, the psychiatrist is being absolutely straightforward in his advice. Derek has told him about two important adverse effects of his medication, and it seems perfectly reasonable for him to want to come off drugs after several years of being well. But the psychiatrist explains the odds of a relapse in blunt terms. This is one area where the opponents of drug treatment have no good arguments to make: however unpleasant the adverse effects of antipsychotic drugs may be in the maintenance treatment of schizophrenia, they do prevent relapse. Derek, of course, can take the plunge and stop his drugs – he cannot be prevented from doing so – but in choosing Scylla over Charybdis, he could prevent diabetes but have a six-week stay in hospital.

The psychiatrist takes an intermediate option of a reduction in antipsychotic medication. This is probably wise. There are many prescribers who adopt the principle of 'if it ain't broke don't mend it' and argue that a fixed dose of medication that has kept a patient well should not be altered. But we have serious adverse effects to contend with; they cannot be ignored. Although stopping medication altogether is likely to lead to relapse, the chances of a setback are much less on a lower dose, and there is no means of knowing what the lowest effective dose actually is. A few lucky patients, like Maria mentioned in the introduction to this book, can calibrate their dosages to their symptoms and adjust her medications accordingly, but in most cases, the time lag between cessation and relapse can be weeks or months.

The third element of importance in this conversation is the frank admission that Derek can stop taking his drugs at any time. There is nothing to stop him apart from taking notice of professional advice. The psychiatrist is just asking him to be honest in his reporting of exactly what he is taking, only for the reason of clarity. If things do go wrong and Derek does relapse, the psychiatrist wants to know exactly what dose of drugs Derek has been taking.

SCENARIO D: THE RECURRENT DEPRESSIVE

Malcolm is a middle-grade manager in a large organisation. He is now aged 55 and is very dissatisfied with his life. He has suffered seven bouts of depression in the last 20 years and has never fully recovered from any of them. He has taken many different antidepressants, beginning with fluoxetine, which helped to some extent but gave him insomnia. He was switched to dothiepin, now called dosulepin, which led to improvement in sleep, but a persistent dry mouth and constipation made him ask for another change. After a period on mianserin and venlafaxine, he finished up on mirtazapine 30 mg daily. But he still feels unhappy about life. None of the tablets has really relieved the depression; they have only given him a different set of side effects. His GP has referred him to a sympathetic female psychiatrist for a complete reassessment.

Doctor:	Hello, Malcolm, I'm pleased to meet you. I realise from the letter I have received that you have had problems for quite some time.
Malcolm:	*(Ruefully)* Yes, I'm becoming a bit of a bore at the GP surgery. I'm always there with the same problem.
Doctor:	Can you just go over it in detail, starting with the first time you first noticed it?
Malcolm:	Golly, that was twenty years ago. It was at a good time in my life. I'd just been promoted at work, I was married two years before and had just had our baby boy. Then I found I couldn't concentrate properly at work and lost all confidence in myself. And to put it bluntly, I've never been completely right since.
Doctor:	*(Gently)* I want you to cast your mind back a bit more. Was there anything that happened about that time that might have triggered off your depression? Or is there a history of depression on your family?
Malcolm:	No, we've always been a very healthy family. When I was growing up, my parents had the idea that anyone who had a mental illness was just not trying hard enough and was making mountains out of molehills. I bet if they were around now, they would say my problem was a molehill.
Doctor:	So was there anything that might have happened at that time that bothered you?
Malcolm:	*(Pausing to think)* I suppose there might have been one thing. When my son was born, my wife was very attached to him and spent a great deal of time playing with him and attending to all his needs. I suppose I felt a little bit out of it.
Doctor:	So were you jealous of your son, for taking the attention away from you?
Malcolm:	Not exactly jealous. I just felt a bit neglected; things that I thought were important and told my wife about didn't seem to have the same impact as before. And then I started questioning my work and whether it was worthwhile. And that's when the cycle of depression came in: 'What am I doing, why am I here, is it all worthwhile?
Doctor:	So in all the years since, what has helped you most to deal with your depression? Has it been one or more of the different tablets you have been taking?
Malcolm:	No, I can't say that the tablets have done any more than take the edge off the depression, to make it tolerable and allow me to cope a bit better?

Doctor:	Can I put my question in a different way? What was the most positive time since you became depressed? Can you put a date on it or say what you were doing?
Malcolm:	Yes I can. I developed a hobby of wood carving and found I was quite good at it. I even won a prize or two at the local village fair. In a funny sort of way, I found I could leave all my worries behind when I was in my shed carving. But I always knew that when I had finished my 'off-duty pastime' as I called it, I would go back to being how I was.
Doctor:	I think we have a clue here. Are you satisfied in your current employment? You mentioned when you were promoted you were very pleased.
Malcolm:	I was then, but not now. When you have been around as a middle manager in a large technology business for as long as I have, you begin to question your purpose. What I do could be done by so many others; it does not require any special abilities. And the final product is way down the line. I don't feel I own it in any way, so I cannot really be proud of my work.
Doctor:	This is not really for me to say, but I get the impression that if you left work and set up a wood-carving business or gallery that you would be much happier than you are now.
Malcolm:	Funny you should say that. I've had the idea myself, but it's just a fantasy.
Doctor:	Why should it be a fantasy? You like wood carving. It makes you feel good. You may or may not need the income – I do not know your personal circumstances – but it seems to me you would be in a happier place if you made the change.
Malcolm:	*(Quite surprised)* Well, well, I wasn't expecting that today. I just thought you'd want to change my antidepressant or something like that.
Doctor:	My feeling is that you have enough antidepressants already. Each of them has a different type of action, so the changes that have been made over the years have some justification. But if they were going to relieve your depression properly, they would have done so by now. I am going to suggest you start reducing your mirtazapine to 30 mg and 15 mg alternate days, and I would like to see you in one month. I also want you to think seriously about a change in your employment. In the longer term, this may be the clue to relieving your depression.

I can hear three cheers of jubilation from Joanna Moncrieff and the critics of psychiatry lobby after reading this account, based on a real conversation. One of the difficulties that afflicts psychiatry today is what I call the groove mentality. Once a pathway in therapeutics is chosen, whether it be psychodynamic psychiatry, behavioural treatments or drug therapy, it tends to be followed to its limits. So the psychiatrist who is well versed in drug treatment and sees a patient with 'resistant depression', as Malcolm's condition is formally described, is determined to follow the psychopharmacology route to more and more different drugs, often in combination, till the patient gives up the battle, irrespective of whether they are better or not.

Switching from one model of mental illness to another is not nearly as common as it should be. In this example, the psychiatrist has switched from the disease model to a social one, recognising from her discussion with Malcolm that the drug route has come to a dead end and there needs to be a change in focus. Switching models is not easy, but if you accept that all of them have a place in treatment, in what I have described as the conjugal model (Tyrer, 2022a), then you can move from one to the other with ease.

What the psychiatrist has recognised is that the only real activity that is satisfying to Malcolm is his wood carving. He is in a rut and needs to be shaken out of it by environmental change. When this is a relatively simple process, it is called social prescribing; when it is more difficult, it is called nidotherapy (www.nidotherapy.com). Whether Malcolm takes up the suggestion of an occupational change is up to him. He may find it difficult; he has spent a grooved existence, and a major change will present challenges, but it could be his salvation.

COMMON FEATURES IN THESE EXAMPLES

The common elements of these scenarios is that there are politeness and respect on both sides, a genuine spirit of open enquiry and acknowledgement of uncertainty. Even if there are arguments about drug prescribing they can be informed ones. The patient knows better than anybody else what it feels like to be mentally ill and to have the positive and negative effects of psychotropic drugs, and the prescriber has greater depth of knowledge about the drugs themselves, their indications and their restrictions, and the dialogue that takes place between them is good for sharing on both sides.

There is another important aspect of the prescribing interview that is not often mentioned by either doctor or patient. It is very common today, and perfectly understandable, for patients to look up their symptoms and their treatment on different websites and write a summary that they present to the doctor at interview. This can be done subtly and indirectly, but if the patient gives the impression that he or she has already got the problem fully sewn up with the solution already found and presented, this is not going to go well.

Doctors and other prescribers are human and like to feel, however unjustifiably, that they have superior knowledge and that it is they who should be dictating the terms of the interaction, not the patients. One of my more cynical colleagues explained it to me in this way; when you have already worked out what the problem is and know the answer you go to see the doctor in a puzzled state, present all the symptoms and ask plaintively, 'What do you think it is, doctor?' As the doctor has already been primed well by your list, the answer is given promptly, and most important, the doctor has made the diagnosis, and his primacy is assured.

There is another secret that most practitioners fail to admit. Very few doctors have any knowledge of even half of the drugs in the last chapter of this book, and those who do know are pharmacologists who rarely treat patients. (The ones in the middle are pharmacists, and they know a great deal more than they are given credit for.) What most practitioners do in practice is prescribe a small number of drugs that they know well and more or less ignore the others unless they are passed on in prescriptions from other doctors. This may seem from the outside to be a very short-sighted practice; surely it is better for doctors to know as many drugs as possible?

But the advantage of this approach is that if doctors give prescriptions for only a few drugs, they tend to get to know each of them very well. The prescribers learn about the best way to calibrate dosage, the likely speed of response and its variability, and they hear about all the adverse effects noted by patients and when over the time of a prescription they occurred. They become experts by prescribing experience, and this knowledge is very valuable when they are advising patients, particularly at the time of initial prescription. If a well-informed patient decides that a certain, probably esoteric drug is the only possible for their condition, they will not only have to overcome the scepticism of the prescriber but also his or her ignorance. In general, it is far better being treated by drugs that are very well known to the prescriber than for both doctor and patient to stride forward in ignorance of their territory. Both are likely to get lost.

I finish this chapter by returning to the patient mentioned in the introduction to this book. In that interview, the doctor was doing extremely well in creating a nocebo response. But now I am assuming that the doctor in the interview has read this book and understand the many errors he made formerly. As a consequence, he has taken more pleasure in his work and has learnt how much more satisfying his interviews have become. This is how he assesses Maureen now. Remember, she is a woman aged 72 who has the idea that the devil is watching her.

Doctor:	Good afternoon, Maureen. I'm Dr Elkington, I'm not sure if we've met before. Sit down and settle yourself, there's no rush. What can I do to help?
Maureen:	*(Nervously)* I think I'm being watched.
Doctor:	That's sounds bothering. Who is it watching you?
Maureen:	I don't know. It might be the devil. He seems to be in the house all the time. He looks like a shadow, but I can watch his lips move, and they are saying things like "your time has come".
Doctor:	That must be very disturbing. Could you describe it in more detail? When does this come on and how does it make you feel?
Maureen:	It's worse in the morning. I have very wild dreams about all sorts of things, and when I wake up, I often see him at the end of the bed wearing a brown tunic with a black cowl. He makes me shudder.
Doctor:	How long has this been going on for?
Maureen:	It started about two months after the neurologist at the hospital diagnosed me with Parkinson's disease and put me on medication. It's called levodopa. It's been very good in taking away my shaking, but it's made me dream more.
Doctor:	So did you ever have this problem – this vision of the devil – before you had the diagnosis of Parkinson's disease?
Maureen:	No, I've never had anything like it before. It's really frightening, makes me not want to go to bed at night.
Doctor:	Has anyone in the family had anything like this or any other mental problems?
Maureen:	No, I come from a nervous family, but nobody has had anything like this before. I'm full of dread waiting to see him, so I can't relax and am awake most of the night.
Doctor:	What is it that concerns you most, Maureen?
Maureen:	*(After a pause, very softly)* Am I going mad?
Doctor:	No, Maureen you are not going mad; I can assure you of that.
Maureen:	I must be mad. Normal people don't see the devil at the bottom of the bed.
Doctor:	There is a very good explanation for this. The tablets you are taking for your Parkinsonism, levodopa, are very good but they do have quite a few side effects, and these include

hallucinations of various kinds. What are called visual hallucinations are ones where your brain sees things that aren't there. That's what levodopa has done. I don't believe that you would have had these hallucinations if you had not taken levodopa.

Maureen: What can I do about it then? I don't want to stop my drugs.

Doctor: There are many other drugs for Parkinson's disease. I will write to your neurologist and suggest he makes a change there. But I am worried about another matter. How long have you been sleeping badly?

Maureen: I was having problems even before I started by tablets. I'm very restless in bed and wake early in the morning feeling terrible.

Doctor: And how do you feel later in the day?

Maureen: It gets better later in the morning, and I often feel quite normal.

Doctor: So when you say you are feeling terrible in the morning, are you also saying you are very depressed at this time?

Maureen: Yes, I suppose I am. I just feel things are hopeless at that time of day.

Doctor: Have you ever felt this way before?

Maureen: No, not exactly. I've had my ups and downs but nothing like this.

Doctor: I think you are abnormally depressed now, and the cause may be your Parkinson's disease. There are several options here, including talking treatments, but if you agree, it would be simplest to take an antidepressant drug called sertraline, at first in a dose of one tablet (50 mg) and if necessary doubling the dose later. You may get some minor side effects such as dizziness and upset stomach, but these tend to wear off quite quickly after a few days. Some people find their sleep is interrupted if they take their medication late in the day, but some find the opposite and find the tablets make them sleepy. So you choose when in the day you take them. You should expect to feel better from your depression within two to three weeks, but you may need longer. People tend to respond more quickly on a higher dose. Once we have a different drug for your Parkinson's disease, we can review how long you need to take the sertraline for. Is all that clear?

Maureen: I think so; it's a lot to take in. But when do you think the devil will leave me alone?

Doctor: Quite soon, I hope. I think your hallucinations of the devil are a combination of the effects of levodopa and your depression. When you are depressed, you only see the bad things in life, and in your case, this is shown by the devil. I would expect to see him gradually disappearing from your life when I see you in three weeks' time.

This interview took a little longer than the unsatisfactory one described earlier, but it was much more productive for both patient and doctor. Two important pathologies have been identified: the hallucinogenic properties of levodopa and the presence of a degree of depression of sufficient severity for treatment. The doctor could have been satisfied with the discovery of the levodopa connection to the appearance of the devil, but he went further and explored the mood disturbance behind it. He also explained the reasons behind the prescription of sertraline and its likely effects in rather more detail than many other doctors would.

COMMON PRINCIPLES IN GOOD PRESCRIBING PRACTICE

I hope that these examples demonstrate a pattern that is relevant to all patient–prescriber interactions. Of course, it is impossible to assume that all interviews can be carried out in this good-natured and informed way. Irritable patients, time pressures, domestic worries, moody doctors and frightening receptionists can all upset this gentle exploration of problems, but there is enough in common in all the examples I have given to extract core elements:

- In a psychiatric consultation more than in a general medical one, neither patient nor prescriber should feel intimidated or that their views are being ignored.
- At an initial interview, when the possibility of drug treatment is mentioned, it should normally be accompanied by a discussion of all treatment options.
- The patient's views about drug treatment need to be ascertained before a decision is made unless the circumstances are such that there is no choice (e.g. rapid tranquilisation).
- Wherever possible, the expected duration of treatment with a drug should be mentioned in the consultation.
- For most drugs, it is wise to discuss the possibility of withdrawal problems whenever a drug is being prescribed. Often this may appear unnecessary, but by now the public is alert to this issue, and it should not be fudged.

- An explanation of the likely course of improvement with drug treatment is necessary to ensure adherence to treatment in both the short and long term.
- In patients taking regular treatment, it is wise to check on the pattern of consumption and any relevant experiences of benefit and detriment.
- When the time comes to stop a drug, the importance of gradual withdrawal should always be emphasised.
- The continued use of psychotropic drugs should be reviewed regularly to prevent unnecessary polypharmacy.
- The prescribing of a psychotropic drug should never be a casual off-shoot from an interview; it is a highly important transaction that needs a serious discussion about its adverse effects, dangers and benefits, as well as its likely duration.
- Neither the patient nor prescriber needs to be a saint to follow this advice. It can be summarised as wisdom laced with common sense, always a useful combination.

We are living at a time when human communication is being devalued by a combination of technology, artificial intelligence and digital substitution, but there is no real substitute for good personal interaction when prescribing a psychotropic drug. This requires the prescriber to reach out to the patient in an open and honest way. Carl Rogers, an admired empathic psychotherapist, put it this way: 'in my relationships with persons I have found that it does not help, in the long run, to act as though I were something that I am not'. So, all of you, follow the Oscar Wilde rule: be yourself, but in the nicest possible way.

MESSAGES FROM CHAPTER 12

1. Never regard the prescription of a psychotropic drug as an optional add-on.

2. Think of the course of drug administration as a journey on a bus or train: you need to know in advance where to get on, how far you have to travel and where you get off.

13

FULL LIST OF PSYCHOTROPIC DRUGS AND THEIR INDICATIONS

When a patient is given a prescription for a drug, the first question likely to be asked after looking at the bottle of tablets is 'What on earth is this unpronounceable name, and what does it tell me to do?' To help answer this question, in this chapter, I list all the drugs used in psychiatric practice by their approved names, their usual dosages, their most common diagnostic indications and their main adverse effects. Many people will know these drugs by their trade names. These are much easier to remember, and pharmaceutical companies take a great deal of trouble in generating them. It is very easy to remember Librium, Valium, Prozac and Viagra so why, you may ask, can we not stick with them? The answer is that these trade names vary from one company to another, and often from one country to another, so it would create confusion if I listed the drugs by these other names. The approved name does not usually change, so it is safest to use this name. It is the approved names that are listed in alphabetical order below.

For most drugs, there is a range of dosage, with the lowest figure the starting dose. 'Divided doses' covers the range between two and four times a day. Patients are usually able to find the right frequency after a few doses.

Acamprosate: Dosage 666 mg three times a day. This drug affects the transmission of GABA, the chemical messenger responsible for calming the body; it has shown some value in reducing craving for alcohol once a person has stopped drinking. It should be given immediately after the subject has stopped drinking alcohol and is normally recommended for one year afterwards.

Agomelatine: Dosage 25–50 mg at night. Mainly used for the treatment of depression but is sometimes used for insomnia as it mimics the effect of the natural sleep-inducing substance melatonin in the

DOI: 10.1201/9781032619019-14

body. May lead to liver disturbance, so avoid in presence of liver disease.

Alprazolam: Dosage 0.5–2 mg for anxiety. Formerly heavily promoted for panic disorder for no good reason. Has a short half-life, leading to clear addiction potential. Readily causes dependence and is specifically excluded for those with personality disorder.

Amantidine: Dosage 100–400 mg daily. A drug used mainly for treating Parkinson's disease but also used sometimes to offset extrapyramidal side effects (EPSEs) with antipsychotic drugs. Should not be stopped abruptly as this can lead to a withdrawal syndrome of confusion, agitation and delirium.

Amisulpride: Dosage 200–800 mg daily (in divided dosage). This is an effective atypical antipsychotic drug. May help with the negative symptoms of schizophrenia (apathy, disinterest, low energy). Sometimes used to prevent nausea after operations.

Amitriptyline: Dosage 10 mg daily, usually at night, for neuropathic pain (neuralgia), 25–75 mg twice daily for depression (or 50–150 mg at night if night sedation preferred). This is toxic in overdosage and has marked anticholinergic side effects (dry mouth, sedation, blurring of vision, difficulty in passing urine, sweating). Can cause a drop in blood pressure when standing up and also lead to sexual difficulties. All these are dose related, and some patients have none of them.

Amobarbital: Dosage 100–200 mg at night for very severe insomnia. Now very rarely used because of addiction risks and death in overdose, so only used in well-supervised settings.

Aripiprazole: Dosage 10–30 mg daily. An atypical antipsychotic drug used for the acute treatment of mania and more regularly in schizophrenic psychoses. A popular drug as fewer extrapyramidal side effects than others. Interacts with SSRIs, so combination avoided.

Asenapine: Dosage 5–20 mg daily. A new atypical antipsychotic which is unusual in being absorbed sublingually (under the tongue). Does not predispose to movement disorders or the metabolic syndrome but can lead to weight gain. Is mainly recommended for hypomanic and manic episodes of bipolar disorder.

Atomoxetine: Dosage 0.5 mg per kilogram to maximum of 120 mg daily. This is an SNRI (selective noradrenaline reuptake inhibitor), but it is not known if this is its mechanism of action in ADHD, its main treatment indication. May reduce appetite and growth rate in children. Best given early in the day as can lead to sleep disturbance.

Benperidol: Dosage 0.25–1.5 mg daily, usually in divided doses. This is a typical antipsychotic drug and so can produce EPSEs in higher doses. Recommended for sexual behaviour disorders but evidence of value very limited.

Bupropion: Dosage 150–300 mg daily. This is an SNRI, originally developed as an antidepressant, but its main use now has been for those who want to give up smoking. Normally given for six weeks only while reducing cigarettes.

Buspirone: Dosage 5–30 mg in divided doses. This is an anti-anxiety drug that is completely free of any dependence potential (see Chapter 7), but it is not as effective as other drugs that have such potential.

Carbamazepine: Dosage between 200 and 1800 mg/day in gradual increasing dosage. Mainly used for treating epilepsy but is also a mood stabiliser, although not as effective as many others.

Cariprazine: Dosage 1.5–6 mg daily in a single dosage. This is an anticonvulsant and an atypical antipsychotic drug used to treat bipolar disorder when lithium is ineffective and is also used for schizophrenic-like psychoses and trigeminal neuralgia. May also be used for alcohol withdrawal but is off label for this use. Although it is atypical, can give rise to EPSEs.

Cetirizine: Dosage 5–10 mg daily. This is one of the non-sedative antihistamines, used mainly for children.

Chloral hydrate: Dosage 430–860 mg (1–2 tablets) at night. Used to treat insomnia but has largely been replaced by other drugs. Often causes upset stomach. Withdraw slowly after repeated use.

Chlordiazepoxide: Dosage 10 mg up to three times daily; maximum 100 mg/day. The earliest benzodiazepine to be used for anxiety. A little less likely to lead to dependence than other benzodiazepines. Frequently used short term in alcohol withdrawal programmes in higher doses, but care should be taken to avoid dependence by withdrawing gradually after repeated dosage.

Chlormethiazole (or clomthiazole): Dosage 192 mg (1 capsule) up to three times daily. Mainly used for insomnia but also for agitation. Maximum of two tablets daily in elderly. Is related to barbiturates but is less prone to dependence, although more prone than chlordiazepoxide. Can also be used in titrated dosage in alcohol withdrawal programmes (initially 2–4 capsules, to be repeated if necessary after some hours: 9–12 capsules daily in 3–4 divided doses on day 1 [first 24 hours], then 6–8 capsules daily in 3–4 divided doses on day 2, then 4–6 capsules daily in 3–4 divided doses on day 3, dose then to be gradually reduced over days 4–6; total duration of treatment no more than nine days).

Chlorpheniramine (chlorphenamine): Dosage 4 mg up to four times daily. Is a sedative antihistamine and therefore a mild hypnotic. Can also be given intravenously for acute allergic reactions.

Chlorpromazine: Dosage very variable: 30–300 mg daily in single or divided doses. This is the original antipsychotic drug. Used in schizophrenia and as a sedative in agitation and severe anxiety. Can produce EPSEs and photosensitivity (so avoidance of sun necessary). Often used in low doses for sedation with significantly fewer side effects.

Cinnarizine: Dosage 15 mg up to three times daily. Is a sedative antihistamine often used to prevent travel sickness but can be used as a mild hypnotic. Can be bought without prescription.

Citalopram: Dosage 20–40 mg daily, less than 40 mg daily in elderly. Is a popular SSRI now recommended for both depression and panic disorder. Leads to withdrawal problems if reduction too rapid after repeated dosage.

Clomipramine: Dosage variable 30–300 mg in divided doses. Is a tricyclic antidepressant but has additional properties that help its effectiveness in obsessive-compulsive disorder as well as depression and some phobic disorders. Has all the adverse effects of amitriptyline (qv). Gradual reduction important, especially after high dosage.

Cloral betaine: see *Chloral hydrate*

Clozapine: Dosage variable beginning with 12.5 mg daily but increasing up to maximum of 450 mg daily. As 1% of patients develop agranulocytosis (loss of white corpuscles in the blood making people very prone to infection), it is necessary in most countries to have regular blood checks and to attend special clozapine clinics. Unlike most antipsychotic drugs, clozapine can elevate mood and be energising. This is the oldest of the atypical antipsychotic drugs and is very atypical as it is unlike any other member. Is used for resistant psychosis when other drugs have failed and also for psychosis linked to Parkinson's disease. Blood levels are altered by cigarette smoking. Can lead to marked constipation and excess saliva production (sialorrhoea).

Dexamphetamine: Dosage 5–60 mg daily, beginning 5 mg twice daily. Used for treatment of ADHD and also for sleep epilepsy (narcolepsy). Needs specialist supervision. If dose too high sleep disturbance, agitation and sometimes paranoia can be shown.

Diazepam: Dosage 2–20 mg daily in divided doses. Diazepam is a very useful drug for emergency treatment, especially for the treatment of repeated epileptic fits (status epilepticus), as without treatment it can be fatal. For this condition, diazepam is usually give directly into a vein using a special formulation (Diazemuls), but even when given by mouth, it is quickly absorbed into the brain. Diazepam is used most often for anxiety in all its forms. It begins to show its effects within 30 minutes. It comes in 2 mg, 5 mg and 10 mg doses, and when reducing benzodiazepines, it is a convenient drug for slow withdrawal. It is well established to be a cause of dependence.

Diphenhydramine: Dosage 25–75 mg daily, tablet or liquid form. This is a popular sedative antihistamine whose action starts within 30 minutes and is taken just before bedtime in the treatment of insomnia. Most often used for motion sickness.

Dosulepin: Dosage 75–150 mg daily. Is a tricyclic antidepressant that is less often prescribed but is effective in the treatment of depression. Common side effects are blurring of vision, constipation and sedation (see *Amitriptyline*).

Dothiepin: see *Dosulepin*

Doxepin: Dosage 75–300 mg daily. This is also a tricyclic antidepressant, used to treat depression but subject to anticholinergic side effects (blurred vision, dry mouth, constipation, drowsiness). Sedation is a very common effect and so taken at night can help insomnia.

Duloxetine: Dosage 60–120 mg daily. This is an SNRI and SSRI used for the treatment of depression and sometimes for neuralgia, especially in neuropathic pain caused by diabetes. Also used for urinary incontinence and is recommended for generalised anxiety disorder. Should be withdrawn gradually.

Escitalopram: Dosage 10–20 mg daily, also available in liquid form. This is a different form of citalopram with the same indications and adverse effects. There is a bit of sleight of hand here. These drugs are fundamentally the same, but the e-form is more active and some claim more effective.

Esketamine: Dosage by intranasal spray, 56 mg on day 1, 56–84 mg twice weekly for weeks 1–4, 56–84 mg once weekly for weeks 5–8, then 56–84 mg every one to two weeks from week 9 onwards. New treatment for depression derived from ketamine, an anaesthetic and analgesic (pain relief). Esketamine acts more quickly than other antidepressants but is a controlled substance, and treatment needs special supervision. Longer-term studies are urgently needed.

Fluoxetine: Dosage 20–60 mg daily, in single or divided doses, preferably not taken at night because of sleep disturbance. Under its trade name, Prozac, fluoxetine introduced the second phase of the psychopharmacological revolution when it was introduced into practice in 1988 as the first selective serotonin inhibitor for depression. It has a long half-life (72 hours), and this makes it less liable to withdrawal problems than many other SSRIs (e.g. paroxetine), but gradual withdrawal is still recommended. Standard adverse effects of SSRIs: nausea, appetite disturbance, anxiety leading to sleep disturbance, vomiting and sexual problems with delayed ejaculation in men. Because it reduces appetite, it is also approved for the treatment of bulimia, an eating disorder. Because it has a long half-life, patients wishing to stop taking SSRIs who have difficulty reducing are sometimes advised to switch to fluoxetine before withdrawal and then to come off fluoxetine gradually.

Flupenthixol (flupentixol): Dosage 3–9 mg daily (for schizophrenic group), 1–3 mg daily (when used for depression). Because this antipsychotic has some energising properties, it can be used for the treatment of depression, and as it has fewer risks of dependence, it might be chosen for those who are dependence prone. Has the same adverse effects as other typical antipsychotic drugs, but these are usually absent in low dosage.

Fluphenazine: Dosage 40–400 mg (higher if given monthly). Most often given as a long-acting injection of fluphenazine decanoate every two to four weeks. Is a typical antipsychotic with the same adverse effects as others, but as drug is long acting in this preparation, they appear later than when given orally. Fluphenazine can also be given by mouth, 2.5–20 mg daily in single or divided dosage and is also available in liquid form.

Fluvoxamine: Dosage 50–300 mg daily. Fluvoxamine is an SSRI used for the treatment of depression and obsessive-compulsive disorders. Has the common side effects of SSRIs (nausea, dizziness, sleep disturbance) and needs to be reduced gradually.

Gabapentin: Dosage 300–3000 mg daily. Gabapentin is an unusual anticonvulsant drug for different forms of epilepsy but is also often used off-label for neuropathic pain, muscle spasticity, anxiety and menopausal symptoms. It is a derivative of GABA, the neurotransmitter involved in generating calm that is simulated by benzodiazepines. There is concern that this group of drugs may be prone to dependence, but the evidence at present is too early to tell.

Guanfacine: Dosage variable by age: 1–4 mg from 6–12 years, up to 7 mg for older children. Guanfacine is licensed for the treatment of ADHD when other stimulants are unsuitable. Sleepiness often an early adverse effect which wears off quickly. Anxiety, appetite reduction and dizziness may be present. No apparent problems in withdrawal.

Haloperidol: Dosage 2–20 mg daily in single or divided doses. Has been the mainstay antipsychotic drug for many years. Used not only in the treatment of schizophrenia but for aggressive behaviour in dementia and personality disorder, in manic episodes in bipolar disorder and in tic disorders and Tourette syndrome. Is also given by intramuscular injection in delirium and when oral medication refused in agitated patients. Has quite marked EPSEs in higher dosage. Also exists in a long-acting injectable form, haloperidol decanoate, dosage 25–150 mg every four weeks, given for the maintenance treatment of schizophrenia.

Hydroxyzine: Dosage: 25–50 mg daily. Hydroxyzine is a standard sedative histamine that can be used for insomnia and does not have the same risks as benzodiazepines, but occasionally abuse can occur.

Imipramine: Dosage 75–200 mg daily, usually in divided doses. Imipramine was the first of the tricyclic antidepressants to be used for the treatment of depression and is still used quite frequently. Has the same adverse effects as amitriptyline but the effect of difficulty in passing urine has a positive use in the treatment of bed-wetting (nocturnal enuresis) in children when only low doses are prescribed.

Isocarboxazid: Dosage 30–60 mg daily, usually twice a day. Isocarboxazid is what is called an irreversible MAOI: it completely stops the action of monoamine oxidase, and therefore, foods high in tyramine (a natural substance that raises blood pressure) are not broken down. Sudden catastrophic rises in blood pressure can occur if foods or drinks with high tyramine content are taken (e.g. matured cheeses such as Stilton and fermented wines such as Chianti). Isocarboxazid is the safest of the MAOIs but has the least value in treating depression and anxiety disorders. It is rarely prescribed now. May also interact with other antidepressants and other drugs. After isocarboxazid is stopped, the dietary restrictions should be continued for at least weeks to allow MAO enzymes to rise to normal levels again.

Lamotrigine: Dosage 25–200 mg daily in divided doses. Lamotrigine is an anti-epileptic drug and a mood stabiliser, so it can be used in the treatment of bipolar disorder. It is one of the few mood stabilisers that is safe to take in pregnancy. Has a range of adverse effects that are usually relatively minor, including agitation, dizziness, drowsiness, dry mouth and sleep problems.

Levomepromazine: Dosage 100–1000 mg daily in divided doses. Levomepromazine is similar to chlorpromazine, but because it is particularly effective in preventing nausea and vomiting and for inducing sleep, it is used mainly for sedation and treatment of nausea, particularly in the elderly. Has the same range of adverse effects as chlorpromazine, but in the dosages normally used in practice, these are not common.

Lisdexamfetamine: Dosage 30–70 mg daily. Lisdexamfetamine is used for the treatment of ADHD under specialist supervision. It can decrease appetite, cause gastrointestinal upsets and lead to nausea and sleep disturbance.

Lithium: Dosage 1–1.5 gms daily, but once stabilised, the dosage is determined by regular checks on blood lithium levels so that these stay within the range 0.6–1.1 mmol/litre. For this reason, regular blood tests are required 12 hours after the last dose. Lithium is used to treat mania (but less often than other drugs), for the maintenance treatment of bipolar disorder, and for the treatment and prevention of aggressive behaviour. It is available in two forms, lithium citrate and lithium carbonate, and there is also a slow-release preparation (Camcolit). Lithium is normally well tolerated but has a range of adverse effects, including gastrointestinal upsets, tremor, and muscle weakness. It often leads to increased frequency of passing urine (polyuria) through its effects on the kidney. It should be avoided in pregnancy. Lithium may also affect thyroid function, so regular monitoring for hypothyroidism is required. If lithium therapy is successful but hypothyroidism develops, thyroid hormones can be prescribed, and lithium can be continued. Lithium has a low therapeutic index of 2, so if blood levels rise above 1.5 mmol/litre, the drug should be stopped immediately. All these problems do not prevent lithium being prescribed long term as a prophylactic (i.e. preventive) treatment in bipolar disorder as it is the most effective mood stabiliser.

Lofepramine: Dosage 140–210 mg daily usually in divided doses. Lofepramine is a tricyclic antidepressant and has the same adverse effects of all of this class of drugs (see *Amitriptyline*) but generally to a lower degree. It is used to treat depression. Gradual withdrawal recommended.

Loprazolam: Dosage 0.5–2 mg at night. Loprazolam is a long-acting benzodiazepine and is used for the treatment of insomnia. It is very similar to the other hypnotic benzodiazepines and is best prescribed as required or very short term. Gradual withdrawal necessary to avoid withdrawal symptoms.

Lorazepam: Dosage 0.5–4 mg daily in divided doses except when used at night for insomnia. This is a potent medium half-life benzodiazepine that is used for more conditions than almost all other benzodiazepines. Because it acts very quickly by intramuscular injection (1.5–2.5 mg up to 6 hourly), it is used to promote aggressive, challenging behaviour and acute severe panic attacks. Its most frequent use is in the treatment of severe anxiety.

Lormetazepam: Dosage: 0.5–1.5 mg taken at night. This is another benzodiazepine marketed for insomnia. It is very similar to loprazolam and has all the characteristics of benzodiazepines, including the need for gradual withdrawal.

Lurasidone: Dosage 37–148 mg daily (odd-sized amounts). Atypical antipsychotic used for schizophrenia group and bipolar disorder.

Melatonin: Dosage 2 mg two hours before bedtime up to 13 weeks. This a natural body drug. When taken to avoid jet lag, 3 mg once daily for up to 5 days, with the first dose taken at the habitual bedtime after arrival at destination except before 8 p.m. or after 4 a.m. The aim is to reshape the sleep cycle temporarily.

Mianserin: Dosage 30–90 mg daily. This is called a tetracyclic antidepressant. It is usually employed as a back-up antidepressant when others fail. Should be withdrawn gradually because of possible withdrawal symptoms.

Mirtazapine: Dosage 15–30 mg at night, occasionally up to 45 mg. This is an antidepressant unlike any other on the market and is often used when standard drugs fail. Care needs to be taken during withdrawal.

Moclobemide: Dosage 150–300 mg daily in divided doses (better after food). This is a reversible MAOI introduced after concern about the previous ones prescribed which are irreversible MAOIs. But patients still have to avoid large amounts of the foods listed with the other MAOIs in this list and also other antidepressants. It is not as effective as the standard MAOIs. It is also used in the treatment of social anxiety.

Nitrazepam: Dosage 5–10 mg at night. Formerly the most commonly prescribed hypnotic under the name of Mogadon. Has a long half-life. Care should be taken regardless withdrawal and is dangerous when taken with alcohol.

Nortriptyline: Dosage 25–150 mg daily, usually in divided doses. Nortriptyline is a tricyclic antidepressant very similar to amitriptyline and has virtually the same beneficial and negative properties. In higher doses, blood levels can be monitored, but the value of this is uncertain. Should be reduced gradually over one to three weeks.

Olanzapine: Dosage 5–20 mg daily. Olanzapine is a very popular atypical antipsychotic that is marketed for the treatment of schizophrenia but is used for bipolar disorder, anorexia nervosa, acute sedation and aggressive behaviour. Its most important adverse effect is to increase appetite (hence its use in anorexia nervosa), but in many patients, this can lead to gross weight disturbance and secondary diabetes. Is best taken when required. May also be given by intramuscular injection in similar doses.

Oxazepam: Dosage 10–40 mg daily in divided doses. Oxazepam is one of the breakdown products of diazepam and is used for the treatment of anxiety disorders. It has all the positive and negative aspects of diazepam and other benzodiazepines and is best taken as required rather than regularly. Should always be reduced slowly.

Paliperidone: Dosage 6–12 mg daily, usually in the morning. Paliperidone is a metabolite of risperidone and is used mainly for the treatment of the schizophrenic psychoses and bipolar disorder. It also exists in a long-acting form, paliperidone palmitate, given once monthly intramuscularly in pre-filled syringes at 100–150 mg or every three months in pre-filled syringes at 175–525 mg. This is often favoured by practitioners. The drug has the advantage that it can be given into the big muscle of the upper arm, the deltoid muscle, whereas most others have to be given into the buttock (gluteus muscle). It has the same adverse effects as most other atypical antipsychotic drugs.

Paroxetine: Dosage 20–50 mg day in variable doses. Paroxetine is a frequently prescribed SSRI for the treatment of depression, but it is also approved for the social anxiety disorder, obsessional disorders, panic disorder and post-traumatic stress disorders. It has a short half-life, and most of the reports of dependence problems with SSRIs have involved paroxetine. Side effects include gastro-intestinal disturbances, headache, anxiety, dizziness and tingling sensations. Withdrawal should be gradual over several weeks.

Periciazine: Dosage 75–300 mg daily, usually in divided doses. Periciazine is a standard typical antipsychotic drug related to chlorpromazine (one of the phenothiazines). Its standard use is for the treatment of psychoses, but it is also used to treat severe anxiety, agitation and disturbed behaviour. It has the same adverse effects as chlorpromazine, including EPSEs.

Phenelzine: Dosage 15–60 mg daily, usually twice a day. Phenelzine is the most commonly prescribed MAOI, but as it is prescribed infrequently, most doctors will not know of it. Is used for the treatment of depression but is most helpful when anxiety and depression are present together, or in severe social anxiety. As other treatments are not especially helpful when mixed anxiety and depression are severe, phenelzine can be considered. However, it has to be given cautiously, and personality assessment (see Chapter 6) comes into deciding when to prescribe. All the food restrictions of MAOIs have to be observed, and it is wise to reduce gradually at the end of treatment.

Pimozide: Dosage 2–20 mg daily, increasing gradually. Used for the treatment of schizophrenic syndromes and what was called monosymptomatic hypochondriacal psychosis (e.g. delusions of parasitical infection) in the past but which is now included under the group heading of delusional disorders. It is not likely to be specific in the treatment of delusional disorders, but several positive case series with pimozide have been reported, so it has achieved a certain eminence.

Pregabalin: Dosage 50–600 mg daily in divided doses. Used as an anticonvulsant but also for the treatment of anxiety (see *Gabapentin*) and generalised anxiety disorder. It may reduce withdrawal symptoms from benzodiazepine reduction and help in maintaining abstinence in alcohol dependence. There is concern that pregabalin, may lead to dependence, but definitive evidence not yet available.

Procyclidine: Dosage 2.5–10 mg daily in divided doses. This is one of the most common anti-parkinsonian drugs used to combat the extrapyramidal side effects of antipsychotic drugs (stiffness, tremor, rigidity). Can be given by injection if these symptoms are severe (acute dystonia). Can cause constipation and urinary retention. Some patients find it has mild euphoriant effects, so it has a black market value.

Promazine: Dosage: 25–200 mg daily, often given every six hours. Promazine is derived from phenothiazines but is seldom used for psychotic disorders. Because it has sedative properties, it is often prescribed to control agitation and severe anxiety.

Promethazine: Dosage 5–50 mg daily in divided doses, or nightly for insomnia. Promethazine is one of the sedative antihistamines used mainly for motion sickness, but it can be used for insomnia.

Propranolol: Dosage 10–40 mg daily in divided doses. This drug is used in higher doses to treat high blood pressure and hypertension, but when used in psychiatry, it reduces heart rate and palpitations and is very effective in reducing tremor, so much so that it is banned for professional snooker players. May cause depression. Avoid in asthma and obstructive airway disease. Reduce gradually.

Quetiapine: Dosage very variable, 25–600 mg daily, starting with low dose; can be given in slow-release form. Atypical antipsychotic used for treating schizophrenia group and bipolar disorder but also as a drug for preventing and treating both depression and bipolar disorder.

Reboxetine: Dosage 4–12 mg daily in divided doses. Is one of the SNRIs but not as widely used as most. Has similar side effects to SSRIs. Gradual withdrawal important.

Risperidone: Dosage 1–6 mg daily. Is an atypical antipsychotic drug for psychosis and bipolar disorder that is also approved for aggressive behavioural problems in children and adults. It raises prolactin levels. Prolactin is a hormone secreted by the brain and is involved in pregnancy and the secretion of milk; when the hormone is unduly raised, it may hinder conception and lead to sexual difficulties. In men, it may lead to galactorrhoea (secretion of breast milk) and enlarged breasts (gynaecomastia). It is best avoided in pregnancy.

Sertraline: Dosage 50–200 mg daily, usually taken once daily when stabilised. Is currently the most prescribed SSRI antidepressant in most countries. Used for the treatment of depression, post-traumatic stress disorder, social anxiety and obsessional disorders.

Has the same adverse effects of other SSRIs but generally is very well tolerated. Needs to be reduced gradually.

Sildefanil: Dosage 50–100 mg one hour before sexual activity. Used for erectile dysfunction. Adverse effects: headache, flushing, dizziness. Avoid in hypertension.

Sodium amytal: see *Amobarbital*

Sodium valproate: Dosage 600–2500 mg daily, usually in divided doses. Is an antiepileptic drug and also a mood stabiliser mainly used in the treatment of bipolar disorder, although it is not as effective as lithium for maintenance treatment. Should be avoided in pregnancy and in women of child-bearing age as the risk of malformations is high.

Sulpiride: Dosage 200–800 mg daily, often taken twice daily. Sulpiride is an atypical antipsychotic drug that is widely used for both the positive (delusions, hallucinations) and negative (apathy, lack of interest and drive) symptoms of schizophrenia. It has mildly stimulating properties that may cause problems in agitated or very anxious subjects.

Tadalafil: Dosage 10–20 mg 30 minutes before sexual activity. Competes with sildefanil for the treatment of erectile dysfunction. Same adverse effects as sildefanil.

Temazepam: Dosage 10–40 mg at night. Temazepam is a benzodiazepine used for the treatment of insomnia. It has abuse potential and should be prescribed short term, and high dosage should be monitored closely. It is essential to withdraw the drug gradually when no longer needed.

Tranylcypromine: Dosage 10–20 mg daily, usually twice daily except when dosage is low. Tranylcypromine is an MAOI with all the handicaps of this group (see *Phenelzine* and *Isocarboxazid*). Dietary restrictions important. Excessive dosage verging on abuse has sometimes been reported.

Trazodone: Dosage 25–200 mg daily. An unusual antidepressant with very different properties from others. It shares some of the properties of antihistamines and so is sometimes used for insomnia and anxiety also. It is a useful back-up drug when others have failed.

Trifluoperazine: Dosage 5–30 mg daily, usually in divided doses. Trifluoperazine is a member of the phenothiazine group of antipsychotic drugs used mainly for psychotic illness in the schizophrenia group. May also be used for severe anxiety in doses up to 4 mg daily, a dose which is normally too low for the standard anticholinergic and parkinsonian side effects to be present.

Trimipramine: Dosage 50–300 mg daily, usually taken at night. Trimipramine is one of the earliest tricyclic antidepressants and is closely related to imipramine. It is probably the most sedating of this group of drugs and is best used for the treatment of depression associated with sleep disturbance. It has the same side effects of other antidepressants and is best withdrawn slowly.

Valproate: see *Sodium valproate*

Venlafaxine: Dosage 75–375 mg daily, usually in divided doses. Venlafaxine is both an SSRI and an SNRI and is often promoted as a stronger antidepressant than others. It is used for the treatment of depression but is also licensed for the treatment of generalised anxiety, panic and social anxiety disorders. It is similar to other antidepressants in its adverse effects, including agitation, gastrointestinal disturbance, dizziness and sedation. Withdrawal is not normally a problem with this drug.

Vortioxetine: Dosage 10–20 mg daily. Vortioxetine is an unusual SSRI that has many other properties. It is used for the treatment of depression and, rather unusually for this group of drugs, it can be stopped immediately as, at least to date, withdrawal effects have not been shown.

Zolpidem: Dosage 5–10 mg at night. Zolpidem is very similar to the other Z-drug, zopiclone, and is also used for the treatment of insomnia. It is recommended for short-term prescription only and needs slow withdrawal.

Zopiclone: Dosage 3.75–7.5 mg at night. Zopiclone is used for insomnia. It was the first of the Z-drugs, and acts in a similar way to the benzodiazepines, to whom they are related. It has the same dependence problems as the benzodiazepines but because they arrived on the scene later, they have less stigma attached. Needs to be withdrawn gradually.

Zuclopenthixol: Dosage 25–200 mg daily. Also given as a long-lasting injection, zuclopenthixol decanoate is given intramuscularly at the test dose of 100 mg, then 200–500 mg every one to four weeks. Has similar adverse effects to flupenthixol decanoate.

The drugs used for dementia are listed in Chapter 11.

ADVANCE TREATMENT DIRECTIVES

People who have had unpleasant reactions with psychotropic, or indeed any other, drugs are able to make advance decisions (sometimes called living wills) about their treatment in the future. For those with severe mental illness who often lack mental capacity at the time they are treated, often in emergency settings, advance decisions may be a way of preventing a repeat of unpleasant drug effects.

An advance decision about treatment can be made by a patient but is likely to be followed more rigorously if it is backed up by a clinician (prescriber) too. It has to be written down, signed by the patient and also signed by a witness. For example, a colleague who is also a patient and has helped in developing NICE guidelines has had brief psychotic episodes. He finds the side effects of haloperidol extremely unpleasant and has given an advance decision that he should not be given haloperidol as an emergency treatment at any time in the future. There is no time limit attached to an advance decision.

REFERENCES

Adams D, Hastings RP, Maidment I, et al. (2023). Deprescribing psychotropic medicines for behaviours that challenge in people with intellectual disabilities: a systematic review. *BMC Psychiatry*, 23, 202.

Agabio R, Saulle R, Rösner S, et al. (2023). Baclofen for alcohol use disorder. *Cochrane Database of Systematic Reviews*, (1), Article No. CD012557. https://doi.org/10.1002/14651858.CD012557.pub3

Al-Haidar FA. (2008). Parental attitudes toward the prescription of psychotropic medications for their children. *Journal of Family and Community Medicine*, 15, 35–42.

Andrews G, Stewart G, Morris-Yates A, et al. (1990). Evidence for a general neurotic syndrome. *British Journal of Psychiatry*, 157, 6–12.

Ashton CH. (2002). Benzodiazepines: how they work and how to withdraw. *The Complete Ashton Manual & Works*. Published online: Benzo.org.uk

Ashton CH, Rawlins MD, Tyrer SP. (1990). A double-blind placebo-controlled study of buspirone in diazepam withdrawal in chronic benzodiazepine users. *British Journal of Psychiatry*, 157, 232–238.

Baldwin DS, Aitchison K, Bateson A, et al. (2013). Benzodiazepines: risks and benefits. A reconsideration. *Journal of Psychopharmacology*, 27, 967–971.

Baldwin DS, Anderson IM, Nutt DJ, et al. (2014). Evidence-based pharmacological treatment of anxiety disorders, post-traumatic stress disorder and obsessive-compulsive disorder: a revision of the 2005 guidelines from the British Association for Psychopharmacology. *Journal of Psychopharmacology*, 28, 403–439.

Balon R, StarcEvic V, Silberman E, et al. (2020). The rise and fall and rise of benzodiazepines: a return of the stigmatized and repressed. *Brazilian Journal of Psychiatry*, 42, 243–244.

Bartlett FC. (1932). Remembering: A study in experimental and social psychology. Cambridge: Cambridge University Press.

Benedetti F, Lanotte M, Lopiano L, et al. (2007). When words are painful: unraveling the mechanisms of the nocebo effect. *Neuroscience*, 147, 260–271.

Bhaumik S, Branford D, Barrett M, et al. (2015). The Frith prescribing guide for adults with intellectual disability (3rd ed.). Hoboken, New Jersey, USA: Wiley/Blackwell.

Bisson JI, Baker A, Dekker W, et al. (2020). Evidence-based prescribing for post-traumatic stress disorder. *British Journal of Psychiatry*, 216, 125–126.

Blackwell B, Mabbitt LA. (1965). Tyramine in cheese related to hypertensive crises after monoamine oxidase inhibition. *Lancet*, 285, 938–940.

Blom-Cooper L, Hally H, Murphy E. (1995). The falling shadow: One patient's mental health care, 1978–1993: Report of the Committee of Inquiry into the events leading up to and surrounding the fatal incident at the Edith Morgan Centre, Torbay, on 1 September 1993. Bloomsbury Publications.

Bonnet U, Scherbaum N. (2017). How addictive are gabapentin and pregabalin? A systematic review. *European Neuropsychopharmacology*, 27, 1185–1215.

Bradley C. (1937). The behavior of children receiving Benzedrine. *American Journal of Psychiatry*, 94, 577–581.

Breggin PR, Cohen D. (2007). Your drug may be the problem: how and why to stop taking psychiatric drugs? Lebanon, IN: Da Capo Press.

Bridler R, Häberle A, Müller ST, et al. (2015). Psychopharmacological treatment of 2195 in-patients with borderline personality disorder: a comparison with other psychiatric disorders. *European Neuropsychopharmacology*, 25, 763–772.

Brijnath B, Xia T, Turner L, et al. (2017). Trends in GP prescribing of psychotropic medications among young patients aged 16–24 years: a case study analysis. *BMC Psychiatry*, 17, 214.

Brindley GS. (1983). Cavernosal alpha-blockade: a new technique for investigating and treating erectile impotence. *British Journal of Psychiatry*, 143, 332–337.

British Medical Journal. (1975). Editorial. Barbiturates on the way out. *British Medical Journal*, 3, 725–726.

Brown TA, Barlow DH. (1995). Long-term outcome in cognitive-behavioral treatment of panic disorder: clinical predictors and alternative strategies for assessment. *Journal of Consulting and Clinical Psychology*, 63, 754–765.

Bullmore E. (2020). The inflamed mind: A radical new approach to depression. New York: Picador.

Busto UE, Bremner KE, Knight K, et al. (2000). Long-term benzodiazepine therapy does not result in brain abnormalities. *Journal of Clinical Psychopharmacology*, 20, 2–6.

Chakos M, Lieberman J, Hoffman E, et al. (2001). Effectiveness of second-generation antipsychotics in patients with treatment-resistant schizophrenia: a review and meta-analysis of randomized trials. *American Journal of Psychiatry*, 158, 518–526.

Clark DM, Salkovskis PM, Hackmann A, et al. (1999). Brief cognitive therapy for panic disorder: a randomized controlled trial. *Journal of Consulting and Clinical Psychology*, 67, 583–589.

Colloca L, Benedetti F. (2005). Placebos and painkillers: is mind as real as matter? *Nature Reviews in Neuroscience*, 6, 545–552.

Cortese S, Adamo N, Del Giovane C, et al. (2018). Comparative efficacy and tolerability of medications for attention-deficit hyperactivity disorder in children, adolescents, and adults: a systematic review and network meta-analysis. *Lancet Psychiatry*, 5, 727–738.

Craske M, Stein M, Eley T, et al. (2017). Anxiety disorders. *Nature Review Disease Primers*, 3, 17024.

Crawford MJ, Sanatinia R, Barrett B. et al. (2018). Lamotrigine for people with borderline personality disorde: a RCT. *Health Technology Assessment*, 22 (17), 1-68.

Cybulski L, Ashcroft DM, Carr MJ, et al. (2022). Management of anxiety disorders among children and adolescents in UK primary care: a cohort study. *Journal of Affective Disorders*, 313, 270–277.

Darker CD, Sweeney BP, Barry JM, et al. (2015). Psychosocial interventions for benzodiazepine harmful use, abuse or dependence. *Cochrane Database of Systematic Reviews*, (5), CD009652.

Daunt R, Curtin D, O'Mahony D. (2023). Polypharmacy stewardship: a novel approach to tackle a major public health crisis. *Lancet Healthy Longevity*, 4, e228–e235.

De Pascalis V, Chiaradia C, Carotenuto E. (2002). The contribution of suggestibility and expectation to placebo analgesia phenomenon in an experimental setting. *Pain*, 96, 393–402.

De Ridder D, Vanneste S, Freeman W. (2014). The Bayesian brain: phantom percepts resolve sensory uncertainty. *Neuroscience & Biobehavioral Reviews*, 44, 4–15.

Denis C, Fatséas M, Lavie E, et al. (2006). Pharmacological interventions for benzodiazepine mono-dependence management in outpatient settings. *Cochrane Database of Systematic Reviews*, 3, CD005194.

Eagles J. (2023). Shrinking to fit. Lincoln: Impspired.

Eardley I. (2013). The incidence, prevalence, and natural history of erectile dysfunction. *Sexual Medicine Reviews*, 1, 3–16.

Elholm B, Larsen K, Hornnes N, et al. (2011). Alcohol withdrawal syndrome: symptom-triggered versus fixed-schedule treatment in an outpatient setting. *Alcohol & Alcoholism*, 46, 318–323.

Fergusson D, Doucette S, Glass KC, et al. (2005). Association between suicide attempts and selective serotonin reuptake inhibitors: systemic review of randomized controlled trials. *British Medical Journal*, 330, 396–402.

Fineberg S, Gupta S, Leavitt J. (2019). Collaborative deprescribing in borderline personality disorder: a narrative review. *Harvard Review of Psychiatry*, 27, 75–86.

Gabriel M, Sharma V. (2017). Antidepressant discontinuation syndrome. *Canadian Medical Association Journal*, 189, E747.

Gaebel W, Salveridou-Hof E. (2023). Schizophrenia and other primary psychotic disorders. In: Tyrer P, editor. Making sense of ICD-11: a guide for mental health professionals. pp. 25–38. Cambridge University Press.

Geddes JR, Burgess S, Hawton K, et al. (2004). Long-term lithium therapy for bipolar disorder: systematic review and meta-analysis of randomized controlled trials. *American Journal of Psychiatry*, 161, 217–222.

Golombok S, Moodley P, Lader M. (1988). Cognitive impairment in long-term benzodiazepine users. *Psychological Medicine*, 18, 365–374.

Gunnell D, Saperia J, Ashby D. (2005). Selective serotonin reuptake inhibitors (SSRIs) and suicide in adults: meta-analysis of drug company data from placebo controlled, randomized controlled trials submitted to the MHRA's safety review. *British Medical Journal*, 330, 385.

Haake M, Muller HH, Schade-Brittinger C, et al. (2007). German Acupuncture Trials (GERAC) for chronic low back pain: randomized, multicenter, blinded, parallel-group trial with 3 groups. *Archives of Internal Medicine*, 167, 1892–1898.

Haddad PM. (2001). Antidepressant discontinuation syndromes. *Drug Safety*, 24, 183–197.

Haddad PM, Nutt DJ. (eds) (2020). Seminars in clinical psychopharmacology (3rd ed.). Cambridge: Cambridge University Press.

Hammond CJ, Niciu MJ, Drew S, et al. (2015). Anticonvulsants for the treatment of alcohol withdrawal syndrome and alcohol use disorders. *CNS Drugs*, 29, 293–311.

Han JS. (2004). Acupuncture and endorphins. *Neuroscience Letters*, 361, 258–261

Hashimoto K. (2019). Rapid-acting antidepressant ketamine, its metabolites and other candidates: a historical overview and future perspective. *Psychiatry & Clinical Neuroscience*, 73, 613–627.

He Q, Chen X, Wu T, et al. (2019). Risk of dementia in long-term benzodiazepine users: evidence from a meta-analysis of observational studies. *Journal of Clinical Neurology*, 15, 9–19.

Hedman-Lagerlöf E, Tyrer P, Hague J, et al. (2019). Health anxiety. *British Medical Journal*, 364, l774.

Horowitz M, Taylor D. (2024). *The Maudsley deprescribing guidelines: Antidepressants, benzodiazepines, gabapentinoids and Z-drugs*. Hoboken, New Jersey, USA: Wiley-Blackwell.

Jones PB, Barnes TRE, Davies L, et al. (2006). Randomized controlled trial of the effect on quality of life of second- vs first-generation antipsychotic drugs in schizophrenia—cost utility of the latest antipsychotic drugs in schizophrenia study (CUtLASS 1). *Archives of General Psychiatry*, 63, 1079–1086.

Kane J, Honigfeld G, Singer J, et al. (1988). Clozapine for the treatment-resistant schizophrenic. A double-blind comparison with chlorpromazine. *Archives of General Psychiatry*, 45, 789–796.

Khin NA, Chen YF, Yang Y, et al. (2011). Exploratory analyses of efficacy data from major depressive disorder trials submitted to the US Food and Drug Administration in support of new drug applications. *Journal of Clinical Psychiatry*, 72, 464–472.

Kingdon D, Turkington D. (1994). Cognitive-behavioral therapy of schizophrenia. New York: Guilford.

Kirsch I, Deacon BJ, Huedo-Medina TB, et al. (2008). Initial severity and antidepressant benefits: a meta-analysis of data submitted to the Food and Drug Administration. *PLoS Medicine*, 5, e45.

Koracevic G, Micic S, Stojanovic M. (2021). By discontinuing beta-blockers before an exercise test, we may precipitate a rebound phenomenon. *Current Vascular Pharmacology*, 19, 6.

Lader M. (2011). Benzodiazepines revisited: will we ever learn? *Addiction*, 106, 2086–2109.

Lader M, Ron M, Petursson H. (1984). Computerized axial brain tomography in long-term benzodiazepine users. *Psychological Medicine*, 14, 203–206.

Lähteenvuo M, Taipale H, Tanskanen A, et al. (2021). Effectiveness of pharmacotherapies for delusional disorder in a Swedish national cohort of 9076 patients. *Schizophrenia Research*, 228, 367–372.

Landgren V, Savard J, Dhejne C, et al. (2022). Pharmacological treatment for pedophilic disorder and compulsive sexual behavior disorder: a review. *Drugs*, 82, 663–681.

Lewis SW, Barnes TR, Davies L, et al. (2006). Randomized controlled trial of effect of prescription of clozapine versus other second-generation antipsychotic drugs in resistant schizophrenia. *Schizophrenia Bulletin*, 32, 715–723.

Lieberman JA, Stroup TS, McEvoy JP, et al. (2005). Effectiveness of antipsychotic drugs in patients with chronic schizophrenia. *New England Journal of Medicine*, 353, 1209–1223.

Lindström L, Lindström E, Nilsson M, et al. (2017). Maintenance treatment with second-generation antipsychotics for bipolar disorder – systematic review and meta-analysis. *Journal of Affective Disorders*, 213, 138–150.

Lingford-Hughes AR, Weich S, Peters L, et al. (2012). BAP updated guidelines: evidence-based guidelines for the pharmacological management of substance abuse, harmful use, addiction and comorbidity: recommendations from BAP. *Journal of Psychopharmacology*, 26, 899–952.

MacKinnon GL, Parker WA. (1982). Benzodiazepine withdrawal syndrome: a literature review and evaluation. *American Journal of Drug and Alcohol Abuse*, 9, 19–33.

Miller FG, Kaptchuk TJ. (2008). Deception of subjects in neuroscience: an ethical analysis. *Journal of Neuroscience*, 28, 4841–4843.

Moncrieff J, Timimi S. (2010). Is ADHD a valid diagnosis in adults? No. *British Medical Journal*, 340, c547.

Moncrieff J. (2020). *A straight talking introduction to psychiatric drugs: The truth about how they work and how to come off them* (2nd ed.). Monmouth, UK: PCCS Books.

Mooney P, Oakley J, Ferriter M, et al. (2004). Sertraline as a treatment for PTSD: a systematic review and meta-analysis. *Irish Journal of Psychological Medicine*, 21, 100–103.

Moran P, Leese M, Lee T, et al. (2003). Standardised Assessment of Personality – Abbreviated Scale (SAPAS): preliminary validation of a brief screen for personality disorder. *British Journal of Psychiatry*, 183, 228–232.

Morrison AP, Pyle M, Gumley A, et al. (2019). Cognitive-behavioural therapy for clozapine-resistant schizophrenia: the FOCUS RCT. *Health Technology Assessment*, 23, 1–144.

Mueller C, Molokhia M, Perera G, et al. (2018). Polypharmacy in people with dementia: associations with adverse health outcomes. *Experimental Gerontology*, 106, 240–245.

Mulder R, Tyrer P. (2023). Borderline personality disorder: a spurious condition unsupported by science that should be abandoned. *Journal of the Royal Society of Medicine*, 116, 148–150.

Murphy SM, Owen R, Tyrer P. (1989). Comparative assessment of efficacy and withdrawal symptoms after 6 and 12 weeks' treatment with diazepam or buspirone. *British Journal of Psychiatry*, 154, 529–534.

Murphy SM, Tyrer P. (1991). The essence of benzodiazepine dependence. In: Lader M, editor. The psychopharmacology of addiction. Oxford: Oxford University Press. pp. 157–167.

Murray RM, Quattrone D, NateSan S, et al. (2016). Should psychiatrists be more cautious about the long-term prophylactic use of antipsychotics? *British Journal of Psychiatry*, 209, 361–365.

National Institute of Care and Clinical Excellence (NICE). (2011). Generalised anxiety disorder and panic disorder in adults: management. London: Department of Health.

Ning AY, Theodoros T, Harris K, et al. (2023). Overdose and off-label psychotropic prescribing in patients with borderline personality disorder: a retrospective series. *Australasian Psychiatry*, 31, 195–200.

Nutt D. (2021). *Drugs without the hot air: Making sense of legal and illegal drugs* (2nd ed.). UIT Cambridge Ltd.

Nutt D. (2023). *Psychedelics: The revolutionary drugs that could change your life – a guide from the expert*. Yellow Kite.

Osler M, Jørgensen MB. (2020). Associations of benzodiazepines, Z-drugs, and other anxiolytics with subsequent dementia in patients with affective disorders: a nationwide cohort and nested case-control study. *American Journal of Psychiatry*, 177, 497–505.

Paloupi E, Ozieranski P, Jones MD. (2023). Professional stakeholders' expectations for the future of community pharmacy practice in England: a qualitative study. *BMJ Open*, 13(1016).

Parry PI, Levin EC. (2012). Pediatric bipolar disorder in an era of "mindless psychiatry". *Journal of Trauma and Dissociation*, 13, 51–68.

Patel DR, Feucht C, Brown K, et al. (2018). Pharmacological treatment of anxiety disorders in children and adolescents: a review for practitioners. *Translational Pediatrics*, 7, 23–35.

Paton C, Crawford MJ, Bhatti SF, et al. (2015). The use of psychotropic medication in patients with emotionally unstable personality disorder under the care of UK mental health services. *Journal of Clinical Psychiatry*, 76, e512–e528.

Petursson H, Lader MH. (1981). Withdrawal from long-term benzodiazepine treatment. *British Medical Journal*, 283, 643–645.

Planès S, Villier C, Mallaret M. (2016). The nocebo effect of drugs. *Pharmacology Research Perspectives*, 4, e00208.

Popova V, Daly EJ, Trivedi M, et al. (2020). Efficacy and safety of flexibly dosed esketamine nasal spray combined with a newly initiated oral antidepressant in treatment-resistant depression: a randomized double-blind active-controlled study. *American Journal of Psychiatry*, 176, 428–438.

Pratt P, Parker C, Khwaja M, et al. (2023). Use of medication and electroconvulsive therapy in the management of violence. In: Khwaja M and Tyrer P, editor. The prevention and management of violence: guidance for mental healthcare professionals (2nd ed.). Cambridge, UK: Cambridge University Press. pp. 75–106.

Price J, Cole V, Goodwin GM. (2009). Emotional side-effects of selective serotonin reuptake inhibitors: qualitative study. *British Journal of Psychiatry*, 195, 211–217.

Radojčić MR, Pierce M, Hope H, et al. (2023). Trends in antipsychotic prescribing to children and adolescents in England: cohort study using 2000–19 primary care data. *Lancet Psychiatry*, 10, 119–128.

Rosenqvist TW, Wium-Andersen MK, Wium-Andersen IK, et al. (2024). Long-term use of benzodiazepines and benzodiazepine-related drugs: a register-based

Danish Cohort Study on determinants and risk of dose escalation. *American Journal of Psychiatry*, 181, 246–254.

Sawan MJ, Moga DC, Ma MJ, et al. (2021). The value of deprescribing in older adults with dementia: a narrative review. *Expert Reviews in Clinical Pharmacology*, 14, 1367–1382.

Schweizer E, Case WG, Garcia-Espana F, et al. (1995). Progesterone co-administration in patients discontinuing long-term benzodiazepine therapy: effects on withdrawal severity and taper outcome. *Psychopharmacology*, 117, 424–429.

Schweizer E, Rickels K, De Martinis N, et al. (1998). The effect of personality on withdrawal severity and taper outcome in benzodiazepine dependent patients. *Psychological Medicine*, 28, 713–720.

Sensky T, Turkington D, Kingdon D, et al. (2000). A randomized trial of cognitive-behavioral therapy for persistent symptoms in schizophrenia resistant to medication. *Archives of General Psychiatry*, 57, 165–172.

Sinclair JM, Chambers SE, Shiles CJ, et al. (2016). Safety and tolerability of pharmacological treatment of alcohol dependence: comprehensive review of evidence. *Drug Safety*, 39, 627–645.

Singh JB, Daly EJ, Mathews M, et al. (2020a). Approval of esketamine for treatment-resistant depression. *Lancet Psychiatry*, 7, 232–235.

Singh S, Roy D, Sinha K, et al. (2020b). Impact of COVID-19 and lockdown on mental health of children and adolescents: a narrative review with recommendations. *Psychiatry Research*, 293, 113429.

Skegg DC, Richards SM, Doll R. (1979). Minor tranquillisers and road accidents. *British Medical Journal*, 1, 917.

Stoffers-Winterling JM, Storebø OJ, Pereira Ribeiro J, et al. (2022). Pharmacological treatment for borderline personality disorder. *Cochrane Database of Systematic Reviews*, 11 (11), CD012956.

Taylor DM, Barnes TRE, Young AH. (2021). The Maudsley prescribing guidelines in psychiatry (14th ed.). Hoboken, New Jersey, USA: Wiley/Blackwell.

Theberath M, Bauer D, Chen W, et al. (2022). Effects of COVID-19 pandemic on mental health of children and adolescents: a systematic review of survey studies. *SAGE Open Medicine*, 10, 20503121221086712.

Tilhonen J, Tanskanen A, Taipale H. (2018). 20-Year nationwide follow-up study on discontinuation of antipsychotic treatment in first-episode schizophrenia. *American Journal of Psychiatry*, 175, 765–773.

Timimi S. (2017). Non-diagnostic based approaches to helping children who could be labelled ADHD and their families. *International Journal of Qualitative Studies in Health and Well-being*, 12(Suppl. 1), 1298270.

Tönne U, Hiltunen AJ, Engelbrektsson K, et al. (1998). Personality characteristics in primary benzodiazepine dependent patients: comparison with controls and poly drug users. *Personality and Individual Differences*, 24, 797–804.

Tournier M, Bénard-Laribière A, Jollant F, et al. (2023). Risk of suicide attempt and suicide associated with benzodiazepine: a nationwide case crossover study. *Acta Psychiatrica Scandinavica*. https://doi.org/10.1111/acps.13582

Tudor Hart J. (1971). The inverse care law. *Lancet*, 297, 405–412.

Tyrer P. (1974). The benzodiazepine bonanza. *Lancet*, 304, 709–710.

Tyrer P. (1976). The role of bodily feelings in anxiety (Maudsley Monograph No. 23). London: Oxford University Press.

Tyrer P. (1978). Drug treatment of psychiatric patients in general practice. *British Medical Journal*, 2, 1008–1010.

Tyrer P. (1980). Dependence on benzodiazepines. *British Journal of Psychiatry*, 137, 576–577.

Tyrer P. (1986). How to stop taking tranquillisers. London: Sheldon Press.

Tyrer P. (1988). Current status of beta-blocking drugs in the treatment of anxiety disorders. *Drugs*, 36, 773–783.

Tyrer P. (2000). A patient who changed my practice: the case for patient-based evidence versus trial-based evidence. *International Journal of Psychiatry in Clinical Practice*, 4, 253–255.

Tyrer P. (2001). The case for cothymia: mixed anxiety and depression as a single diagnosis. *British Journal of Psychiatry*, 179, 191–193.

Tyrer P. (2002). Nidotherapy: a new approach to the treatment of personality disorder. *Acta Psychiatrica Scandinavica*, 105, 469–471.

Tyrer P. (2008). So careless of the single trial. *Evidence-Based Mental Health*, 11, 65–66.

Tyrer P. (2010). Benzodiazepine substitution for dependent patients: going with the flow. *Addiction*, 105, 1875–1876.

Tyrer P. (2012). From the Editor's Desk. *British Journal of Psychiatry*, 201, 168.

Tyrer P. (2022a). Models for mental disorder, and why the conjugal model is best (6th ed.). Lincoln: Impspired.

Tyrer P. (2022b). Neurosis: understanding common mental illness. Cambridge: Cambridge University Press.

Tyrer P, Alexander J. (1979). Classification of personality disorder. *British Journal of Psychiatry*, 135, 163–167.

Tyrer P, Silk K. (eds) (2008). *Cambridge Textbook of Effective Treatments in Psychiatry*. Cambridge: Cambridge University Press.

Tyrer P, Silk K. (2011). *Effective Treatments in Psychiatry*. Cambridge: Cambridge University Press.

Tyrer P, Alexander MS, Cicchetti D, et al. (1979). Reliability of a schedule for rating personality disorders. *British Journal of Psychiatry*, 135, 168–174.

Tyrer P, Ferguson B, Hallstrom C, et al. (1996). A controlled trial of dothiepin and placebo in treating benzodiazepine withdrawal symptoms. *British Journal of Psychiatry*, 168, 457–461.

Tyrer P, Gardner M, Lambourn J, et al. (1980). Clinical and pharmacokinetic factors affecting response to phenelzine. *British Journal of Psychiatry*, 136, 359–365.

Tyrer P, Mulder R, Kim Y-R, et al. (2019). The development of the ICD-11 classification of personality disorders: an amalgam of science, pragmatism and politics. *Annual Review of Clinical Psychology*, 15, 481–502.

Tyrer P, Murphy S, Riley P. (1990). The benzodiazepine withdrawal symptom questionnaire. *Journal of Affective Disorders*, 19, 53–61.

Tyrer P, Oliver-Africano PC, Ahmed Z, et al. (2008). Risperidone, haloperidol and placebo in the treatment of aggressive challenging behaviour in intellectual disability: randomized controlled trial. *Lancet*, 371, 55–61.

Tyrer P, Owen R, Dawling S. (1983). Gradual withdrawal of diazepam after long-term therapy. *Lancet*, 321, 1402–1406.

Tyrer P, Rutherford D, Huggett T. (1981). Benzodiazepine withdrawal symptoms and propranolol. *Lancet*, 317, 520–522.

Tyrer P, Seivewright N, Murphy S, et al. (1988). The Nottingham study of neurotic disorder: comparison of drug and psychological treatments. *Lancet*, 332, 235–240.

Tyrer P, Tyrer H, Johnson T, et al. (2022). Thirty year outcome of anxiety and depressive disorders and personality status: comprehensive evaluation of mixed symptoms and the general neurotic syndrome in the follow-up of a randomized controlled trial. *Psychological Medicine*, 52, 3999–4008.

Tyrer PJ, Lader MH. (1974). Response to propranolol and diazepam in somatic and psychic anxiety. *British Medical Journal*, 2, 14–16.

Vasant DH, Paine PA, Black CJ, et al. (2021). British Society of Gastroenterology guidelines on the management of irritable bowel syndrome. *Gut*, 70, 1214–1240.

Vikander B, Koechling UM, Borg S, et al. (2010). Benzodiazepine tapering: a prospective study. *Nordic Journal of Psychiatry*, 64, 273–282.

von Buedingen F, Hammer MS, Meid AD, et al. (2018). Changes in prescribed medicines in older patients with multimorbidity and polypharmacy in general practice. *BMC Family Practice*, 28, 19, 131.

Whittington CJ, Kendall T, Fonagy P, et al. (2004). Selective serotonin reuptake inhibitors in childhood depression: systematic review of published versus unpublished data. *Lancet*, 363, 1341–1345.

Wojnowski NM, Zhou E, Jee YH. (2022). Effect of stimulants on final adult height. *Journal of Pediatric and Endocrinological Metabolism*, 35, 1337–1344.

INDEX

Note: Page numbers in *italics* indicate a figure and page numbers in **bold** indicate a table on the corresponding page.

Printed in the United States
by Baker & Taylor Publisher Services